Strategies in Fracture Treatments

Series editors

Peter Biberthaler
Klinik u. Poliklinik für Unfallchirurgie
TU München Klinikum rechts der Isar
München, Bayern, Germany

James P. Waddell
St. Michael's Hospital
Toronto, Canada

This series provides a clearly structured and comprehensive overview of fracture treatments based on the most recent scientific data. Each book in the series is organized anatomically, so the surgeon can quickly access practical aspects, examples, pearls and pitfalls of specific areas. Trauma and orthopaedic surgeons worldwide who are searching for a current knowledge of new implants, therapeutic strategies and advancements will be able to quickly and efficiently apply the information to their daily clinical practice. The books in the series are written by a group of experts from the Association for the Rationale Treatment of Fractures (ARTOF) who aim to provide an independent, unbiased summary of fracture treatments to improve the clinical and long term outcomes for patients.

More information about this series at http://www.springer.com/series/13623

Peter Biberthaler • Sebastian Siebenlist
James P. Waddell
Editors

Acute Elbow Trauma

Fractures and Dislocation Injuries

Springer

Editors
Peter Biberthaler
Department of Trauma Surgery
Technical University Munich
Klinikum rechts der Isar
Munich
Germany

James P. Waddell
St. Michael's Hospital
Toronto
ON
Canada

Sebastian Siebenlist
Department of Orthopaedic
Sports Medicine
Technical University Munich
Klinikum rechts der Isar
Munich
Germany

ISSN 2364-8295 ISSN 2364-8309 (electronic)
Strategies in Fracture Treatments
ISBN 978-3-319-97848-2 ISBN 978-3-319-97850-5 (eBook)
https://doi.org/10.1007/978-3-319-97850-5

Library of Congress Control Number: 2018960385

This Springer imprint is published by the registered company Springer Nature Switzerland AG
The registered company address is: Gewerbestrasse 11, 6330 Cham, Switzerland

Preface

The main therapeutic target of complex elbow trauma is a narrow path between stiffness and instability. In this regard, the elbow joint is one of the anatomic regions that saw the biggest changes in therapeutic concepts during the last decade. Over a long period, this joint was recognized as "the forgotten" joint since its complexity of bony and soft tissue structures orchestrating a highly sophisticated mobility concept of flexion/extension and pro-/supination overstrained the armamentarium of classical surgical implant technologies. Hence, a functional bow of flexion/extension between 30° and 130° was described as a sufficient therapeutic target tipping the scales towards stiffness. Due to the intensive research of several dedicated surgeons and the development of several highly specific implant series, therapeutic options were significantly improved during the last decade. Moreover, the thorough understanding of soft tissue structures and their contribution to elbow joint function induced a whole series of new surgical techniques to stabilize complex elbow injuries sufficiently. This approach allowed to control the instability problem more and more and extended the posttraumatic function consecutively towards a more and more original functional ability.

Hence, the intention of this book was to gather those innovative technologies in a comprehensive piece of knowledge. It is clear that such an ambitious goal can only be achieved by the concentrated work of leading international experts. Therefore, I would like to express my deep thanks to all authors of this book who shared their precious knowledge with the reader to the benefit of our patients.

This book is part of the ARTOF (Association for the rational treatment of fractures) trauma series published by Springer Nature. ARTOF (www.artof-online.org) is an independent scientific society dedicated to a strict scientific approach of the best therapeutic concept of fractures.

More volumes are

Proximal Humerus Fractures

Fractures Around the Knee

Munich, Germany	Peter Biberthaler
Munich, Germany	Sebastian Siebenlist
Toronto, ON, Canada	James P. Waddell
January 2019	

Contents

Contributors

Arne Berner Center for Muskuloskeletal Surgery, Charite – University Medicine, Berlin, Germany

Peter Biberthaler Department of Trauma Surgery, University Hospital Rechts der Isar, Technical University Munich, Munich, Germany

Karl Braun Department of Trauma Surgery, University Hospital Rechts der Isar, Technical University Munich, Munich, Germany

Arne Buchholz Clinic for Trauma Surgery, University Hospital Klinikum Rechts der Isar, Technical University, Munich, Germany

Klaus J. Burkhart Arcus Sportklinik, Pforzheim, Germany

Moritz Crönlein Department of Trauma Surgery, Klinikum rechts der Isar, Munich, Germany

Stephan Deiler Interdicsiplinary Center of Hands (IHZ), Clinic and Polyclinic for Trauma Surgery and Orthopedics, Munich, Germany

Hans-Henning Eckstein Department of Vascular and Endovascular Surgery, Klinikum rechts der Isar, Technical University of Munich, Munich, Germany

Markus A. E. Gühring Klinik im Kronprinzenbau, Reutlingen, Germany

Michael Hackl Department of Orthopedic and Trauma Surgery, University Hospital of Cologne, Cologne, Germany

Jeremy Alan Hall University of Toronto, Toronto, ON, Canada

Andreas B. Imhoff, MD Orthopaedic Surgery and Traumatology, Department of Orthopaedic Sports Medicine, Hospital Rechts der Isar, University of Munich, Munich, Germany

Graham J. W. King, MD, MSc, FRCSC Roth McFarlane Hand and Upper Limb Centre, St. Joseph's Health Centre, Western University, London, ON, Canada

Andreas Lenich Helios Klinikum München West, Department for Orthopeadic-, Trauma-, Hand- and Sportorthopeadic Surgery, München, Germany

Martin Lucke Surgical Clinic Munich South, Munich, Germany

Lars Peter Müller Department of Orthopedic and Trauma Surgery, University Hospital of Cologne, Cologne, Germany

Michael Leopold Nerlich Department of Trauma Surgery, University Medical Center, Regensburg, Germany

Benedikt Reutersberg Department of Vascular and Endovascular Surgery, Klinikum rechts der Isar, Technical University of Munich, Munich, Germany

Gunter H. Sandmann Department of Trauma Surgery, University Hospital Rechts der Isar, Technical University Munich, Munich, Germany

Sportklinik Ravensburg, Ravensburg, Germany

Sebastian Siebenlist Department of Orthopaedic Sports Medicine, Technical University Munich Klinikum rechts der Isar, Munich, Germany

Ulrich Stöckle Berufsgenossenschaftliche Unfallklinik Tübingen, Tübingen, Germany

Jason A Strelzow, MD, FRCSC Department of Orthopaedic Surgery and Rehabilitation Medicine, University of Chicago, Chicago, Illinois, USA

Helen Vester Interdicsiplinary Center of Hands (IHZ), Clinic and Polyclinic for Trauma Surgery and Orthopedics, Munich, Germany

James P. Waddell St. Michael's Hospital, Toronto, ON, Canada

Kilian Wegmann Department of Orthopedic and Trauma Surgery, University Hospital of Cologne, Cologne, Germany

Heiko Wendorff, FEBVS Department of Vascular and Endovascular Surgery, Klinikum rechts der Isar, Technical University of Munich, Munich, Germany

Simple Elbow Dislocations

1

Sebastian Siebenlist and Peter Biberthaler

Epidemiology

Regarding major human joints, the elbow is the second most commonly dislocated joint in adults following the shoulder [1]. By definition, a simple elbow dislocation is described as one without concomitant fractures (apart from small periarticular bony avulsions of 1 mm or 2 mm in diameter) [2]. Several authors reported on the incidence of simple elbow dislocations ranging from 3 to 9 per 100.000 individuals referred to different periods of life [1, 3–5]. Male adults are the group at highest risk. They are more likely to suffer from an elbow dislocation injury following sports or accidents. Women are likely to suffer from dislocations during a fall from standing height with daily activities.

Over the last decades, good functional outcomes have been reported after non-operative treatment in most patients. However, a small proportion of patients complains of recurrent instability, stiffness or pain if treated non-operatively and do require operative intervention in the sequel [3, 6, 7]. Due to better understanding of injury patterns and developments in soft tissue repair techniques the discussion of standard treatment for simple elbow dislocation has arisen again in recent years [8].

Classification

To this day, no validated classification exists for simple elbow dislocations. There is consensus to descriptively grade the injury according to the direction of dislocated forearm related to the humerus (Fig. 1.1). The most common direction of elbow dislocation is posterior and posterolateral respectively. Divergent and anterior dislocations are extremely rare and usually occur in paediatrics or in association with concomitant fractures.

In newer times, the complex interactions among the different elbow stabilizers have been better understood due to improvements of biomechanical knowledge, and therefore current surveys deal with systemizing this "simple" injury [9, 10]. An exhaustive and practical classification is still highly difficult to create because numerous and different parameters are to be considered. However, eminent elbow surgeons have described the elbow instability based on the following criteria: timing (acute, chronic, recurrent), injured ligaments and soft tissues, articulations involved (radio-ulno/humeral or proximal radioulnar),

S. Siebenlist (✉)
Department of Orthopaedic Sports Medicine, Technical University Munich Klinikum rechts der Isar, Munich, Germany
e-mail: sebastian.siebenlist@tum.de

P. Biberthaler
Department of Trauma Surgery, University Hospital Rechts der Isar, Technical University Munich, Munich, Germany
e-mail: Peter.Biberthaler@mri.tum.de

P. Biberthaler et al. (eds.), *Acute Elbow Trauma*, Strategies in Fracture Treatments,
https://doi.org/10.1007/978-3-319-97850-5_1

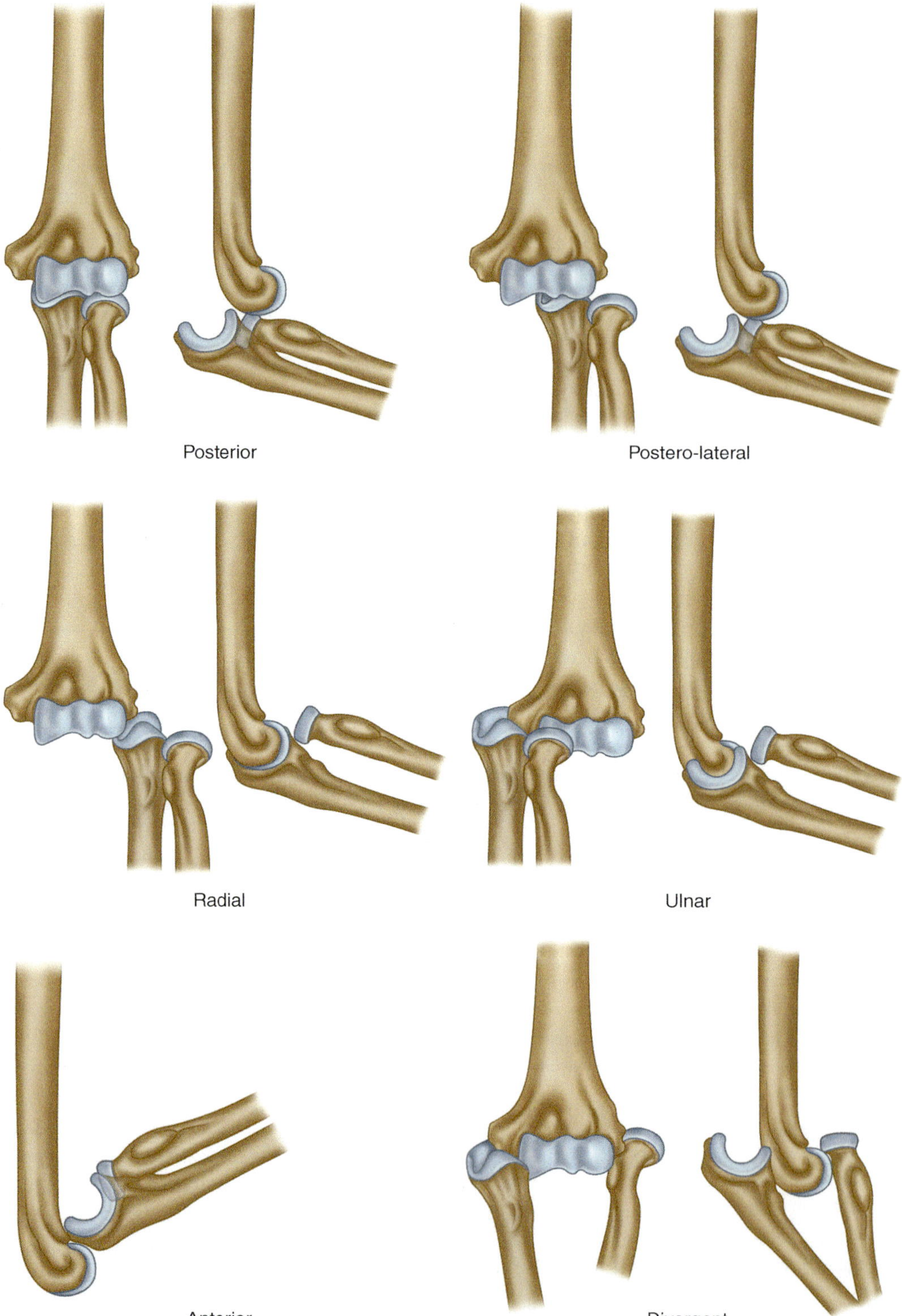

Fig. 1.1 Directions of elbow dislocation

direction (valgus, varus, anterior, posterolateral), degree (subluxated, perched, dislocated) and according to associated fractures (radial head, coronoid, olecranon, distal humerus) [11–15].

Symptoms and Diagnostics

With special respect to the mechanism of injury a detailed case history interview and an accurate physical examination should be performed. In most cases the history gives a lead to the diagnosis. However, the dislocation mechanism (arm position at time of impact) has to be determined as precisely as possible to receive information about the dislocation pattern (→ *subchapter injury pattern!*). Some patients report self- or spontaneous reduction and just complain about pain and swelling, but no deformity. These patients should be exactly interviewed about a history of a clicking event, deformity at the time of injury or a feeling of elbow instability. The elbow has to be evaluated for open wounds as well as for neurologic or vascular disturbances that are described in rare cases [16].

Patients with a dislocated joint at time of presentation frequently report strong pain in the elbow in a typically, slightly flexed position. Prior to reduction, anteroposterior and lateral radiographs are performed to confirm dislocation, to determine direction of dislocation and to exclude associated fractures as well. If the diagnosis is confirmed an immediate closed reduction should be performed by using a gentle reduction maneuver [17]. Subsequently the elbow is immobilized in a posterior plaster cast (→ *subchapter non-operative treatment!*). Again the postreduction neurovascular examination is mandatory and has to be documented. Following reduction radiographs have to be reviewed for joint congruency and to rule out previously unrecognized, concomitant fractures. A CT scan can be necessary for questionable associated fractures or bony avulsions (especially at the coronoid tip!).

During the next days after reduction the physical evaluation should focus on medial or lateral bruising after removing any cast or dressing. An edema and hematoma formation medially and/or

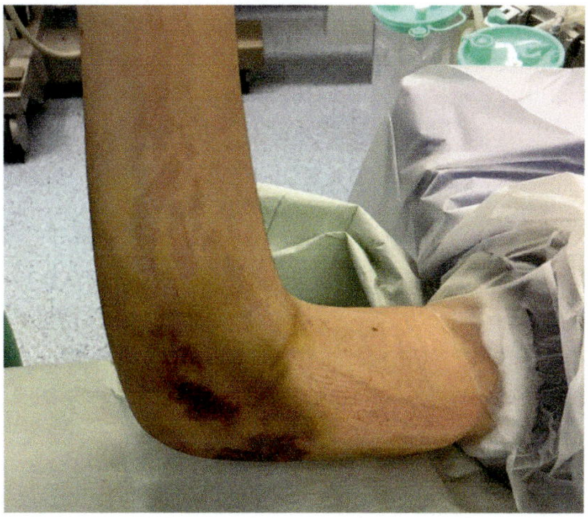

Fig. 1.2 The massive hematoma at the medial elbow indicates an extensive soft tissue injury (disruption of the flexor mass and muscular fascia) following simple dislocation

laterally points to an extensive soft tissue disruption including the tough muscular fascia (Fig. 1.2). In the acute injury the stress testing for ligament integrity is very often not sufficiently feasible due to pain inhibition. In any case the patient should be instructed to actively move his elbow to verify muscular joint centering and stabilization (→ *subchapter injury pattern!*). In the author's experience a reluctance to actively move the injured elbow is highly suspicious of a grossly joint instability based on substantial soft tissue injury. Many of these patients also describe apprehension of recurrent dislocation. Finally, the examination should also include the ipsilateral shoulder and wrist not to miss further injuries.

Anteroposterior and lateral radiographs should be repeated within the first week after reduction to secure a concentric reduction. An initial drop sign (= ulnohumeral distance >3–4 mm) caused by effusion has to be diminished within this time. Otherwise reasons for its persistence like incarcerated ligamentous tissue or loose cartilage bodies have to be detected [18].

Not only for that reason, a MRI examination (ideally obtained within the first week post injury) has to be recommended after any simple elbow dislocation. Using MRI scans Hackl et al.

specified cutoff points for radiocapitellar incongruity and axial ulnohumeral incongruity in patients with posterolateral rotatory instability [19]. To provoke joint incongruencies it is crucial to perform the MRI examination in the nearly extended elbow. Only then the MRI illustrates the integrity of the static ligamentous constraints and of the dynamic muscular stabilizers as well (→ *subchapter injury pattern!*). The MRI scans therefore should be screened with special respect to the lateral ligament complex (LCL), the anterior bundle of the medial collateral ligament (MCL), the flexor–pronator origin, and the common extensor origin (Figs. 1.3 and 1.4). However, it has to be clearly stated that the MRI findings should not be overemphasized and have be assessed in relation to the whole clinical presentation.

Ultrasound examination can also provide valuable additional information when analyzing the collateral ligaments and the common flexor and extensors by dynamic testing. Nevertheless, especially in the acute injury this examination is heavily dependent on the patient's pain, swelling and compliance, but principally on the surgeon's experience.

Also, the fluoroscopy is valuable to dynamically assess the elbow under varus and valgus stress (in full extension and 30° of flexion) and to visualize the degree of stable functional arc. Some authors prefer the fluoroscopy to determine joint stability and to justify their treating protocol for nonsurgical or surgical management [20, 21]. In the anteroposterior view, the angle between the distal humeral joint line and the proximal ulnoradial joint line is measured under maximal varus and valgus stress. It seems probable that the bigger this angle can be opened during examination the more severe is the damage of soft tissue stabilizers on the medial and/or the lateral side (Fig. 1.5). This hypothesis is underlined by a current study of Adolfsson et al. showing that vast soft tissue injuries including both collateral ligaments and muscle origins lead to redislocation in nonsurgically treated simple elbow dislocations [22]. Consequently, it is obvious that an elbow that redislocates under fluoroscopic examination needs surgical intervention due to gross instability. The examination is ideally performed under anesthesia at time of reduction. However, the evaluation of stability using fluoroscopy requires adequate experience in elbow disorders management.

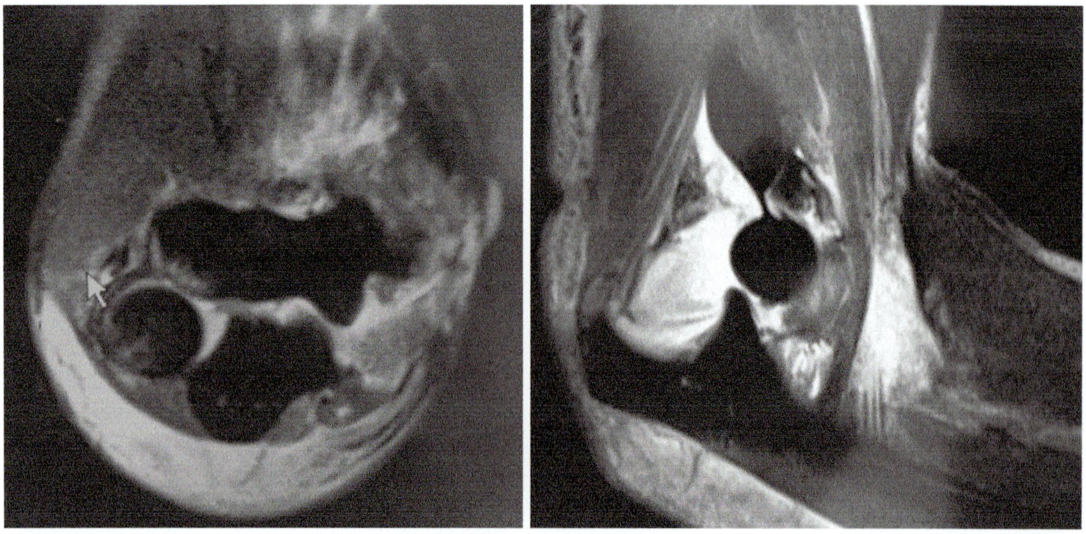

Fig. 1.3 51-year-old male patient after skiing accident: MRI showing re-dislocation of the elbow joint within the applied plaster cast. The brachialis muscle and the flexor-pronator-mass are totally ruptured

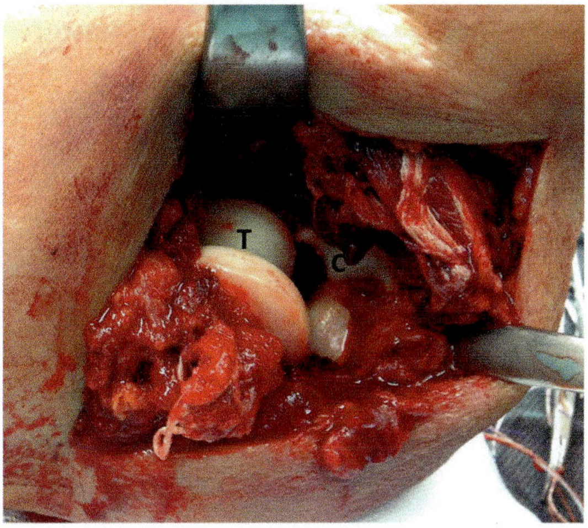

Fig. 1.4 Intraoperative situs of patient presented in Fig. 1.3: following skin incision at the medial elbow it's obvious that all soft tissue stabilizers (MCL complex, flexor-pronator mass and brachialis muscle) are stripped of the humerus (*T* humeral trochlea, *C* coronoid)

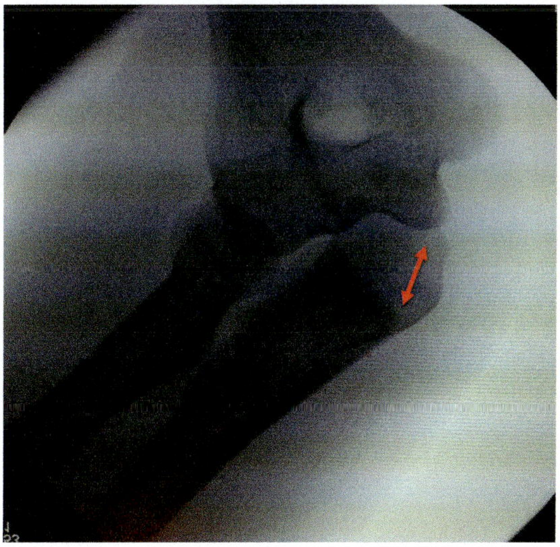

Fig. 1.5 Medial stability testing using fluoroscopy: a grossly openable joint (red arrow) point to severe damage of soft tissue stabilizers

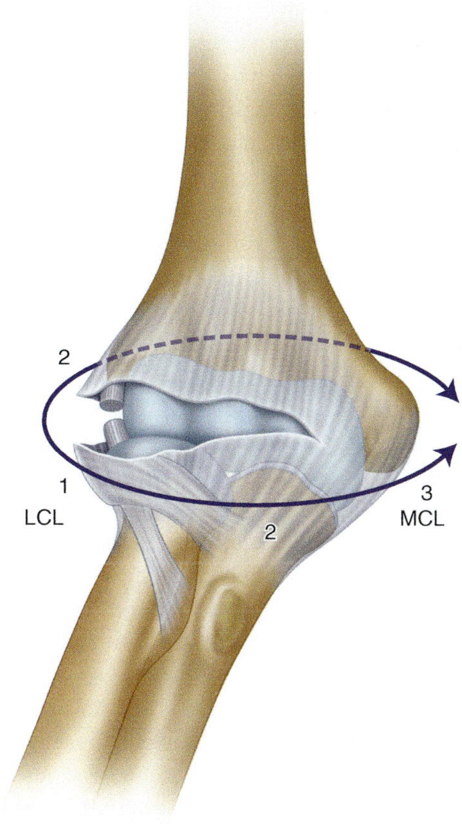

Fig. 1.6 The stages of 'Horii circle':
Stage 1: the partial or complete disruption of the LUCL on the lateral side results in posterolateral rotatory subluxation.
Stage 2: the disruption of the capsule both anteriorly and posteriorly leads to incomplete posterolateral dislocation.
Stage 3A: all the soft tissues except the anterior bundle of the MCL are disrupted. This leads to posterior dislocation of the elbow with pivoting around the MCL.
Stage 3B: the entire medial ligament complex is disrupted.
Stage 3C: the entire distal humerus is stripped of soft tissues including the flexor–pronator mass

Injury Pattern and Surgery Related Anatomy

The exact mechanism of elbow dislocation injuries is still the subject of debate in the current literature. The proposed posterolateral rotation theory of Shawn O'Driscoll – named the 'Horii circle' – is the most cited and accepted injury pattern (Fig. 1.6) [23, 24]. He described a soft tissue disruption from lateral to medial caused by a fall onto the outstretched hand. The soft tissue disruption subsequently results due to co-occuring of valgus, axial and supination forces while the elbow is reflexively flexed when the hand hits the ground. Starting from the lateral side the LCL is ruptured and then proceeds via the capsule to the MCL being injured last. Nevertheless, in some cases the MCL remains intact.

By contrast, an isolated massive valgus moment is also thought to be responsible for elbow dislocation [25, 26]. Recently published studies postulate the progression of soft tissue injury from the medial to the lateral side with an initial rupture of the MCL. Following MCL rupture the flexor-pronator mass disrupts, induced by a sudden distraction; thereby the coronoid becomes disengaged and the radiocapitellar joint dislocates with a pathological forearm external rotation, causing radiocapitellar bone contusion and stripping of the lateral soft tissues from the humerus and ending in posterolateral dislocation (Fig. 1.7) [21]. As the characteristic deforming force a valgus moment with an axial load and progressive supination is often described [27–29]. Own clinical practice confirm this theory as we often see isolated MCL disruptures with simultaneous medial muscular-fascial laceration following dislocation (Fig. 1.8).

In simple elbow dislocations, the osseous integrity is not compromised by definition. Therefore, both static and dynamic soft tissue stabilizers have to maintain elbow stability [30]. Static constraints comprise the LCL, the MCL and the capsule as well. The LCL as the primary constraint to external rotation and varus stress is separated in three components, the lateral ulnar collateral ligament (LUCL), the radial collateral ligament (RCL) and the annular ligament (AL) (Fig. 1.9a). Mainly the LUCL provides varus and posterolateral stability. Stripping offthe complete lateral ligament complex (further RCL and AL) results in posterior subluxation of the radial head [31].

The MCL consisting of the anterior and posterior bundle (Fig. 1.9b) plays the key role in valgus and posteromedial stability of the elbow. The anterior bundle as the "*guiding bundle* "stabilizes against valgus stress during flexion; the posterior part equally contributes at 120° of flexion and resists posteromedial movements [32]. The anterior capsule is furthermore postulated as valgus stabilizer.

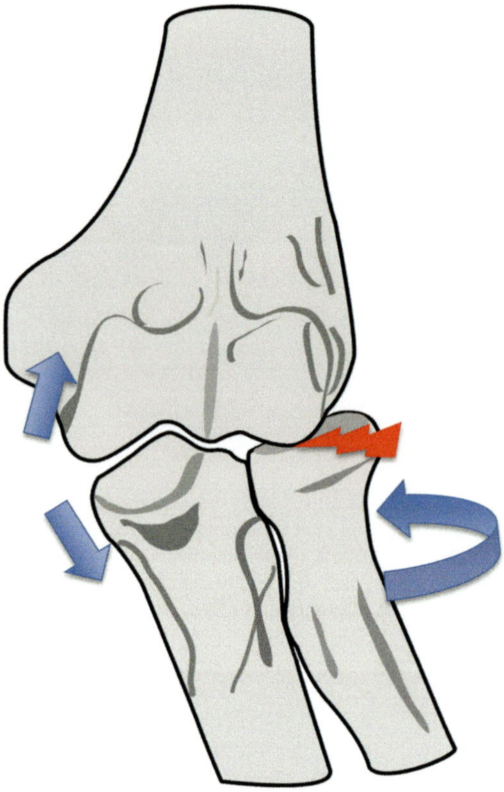

Fig. 1.7 Medial disruption injury mechanism: During valgus stress forces the injury cascade begins medially by disrupting the medial soft tissues (MCL and flexor–pronator origin) in a distractive type mechanism. The capsule is pulled off the coronoid process and the radiocapitellar joint dislocates with a pathological forearm external rotation, stripping off the lateral soft tissues from the humerus, ending in posterolateral dislocation

According to Adolfsson et al. patients with simple elbow dislocations routinely have disruption of both the MCL and LCL and the capsule, but joint stability is still provided in most of the patients by the intact forearm musculature originating on the epicondyles [22]. The dynamic stabilizing effect of these muscles from the common extensor origin (CEO) and the common flexor-pronator origin (CFO) is quite often underestimated. Both muscle masses serve as very important secondary constraints against varus and valgus stress depending on the degree of flexion [33]. The anconeus muscle is also presumed to dynamically resist against varus and posterolateral shear forces [34]. The muscles that cross the elbow joint (biceps, triceps and brachialis muscle) additionally provide dynamic stabilization throughout joint compression, especially if the static stabilizers have been injured.

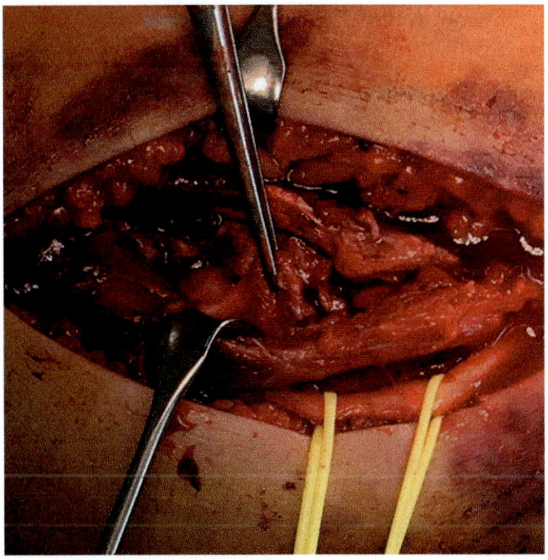

Fig. 1.8 Intraoperative situs of patient presented in Fig. 1.2: Medial disruption of flexor-pronator mass and MCL (forceps) following simple elbow dislocation (yellow loops = ulnar nerve)

Moreover, forearm rotation plays an important role in elbow stabilization especially in the presence of injury. King and colleagues have shown that pronation will stabilize the LCL-deficient elbow while supination decreases stability in the dislocation injury setting [35]. Correspondingly supination stabilises the MCL-deficient elbow [36]. The combined tendon of the flexor-pronator mass can develop its maximal stabilizing potential when the forearm is supinated; the CEO muscles have maximal tension in full pronation and can therefore most effectively act as varus stabiliser [37]. These effects are used for nonsurgical or postoperative treatment protocols.

Therapeutic Options

Non-operative Treatment

Most of the patients with simple elbow dislocations can be treated non-operatively following closed joint reduction and complete evaluation of stability (*→ subchapter symptoms and diagnostics!*). If the elbow cannot be closely reducted

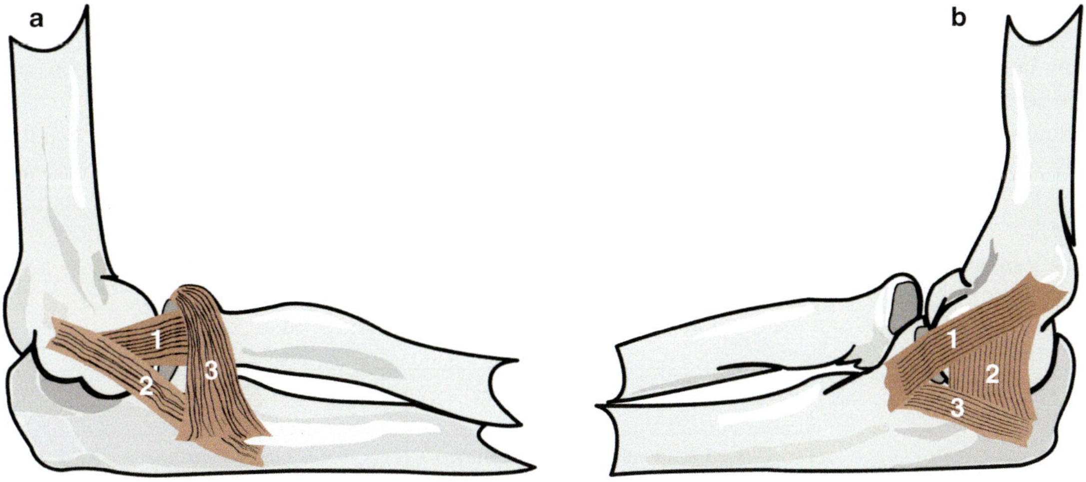

Fig. 1.9 (**a**) The lateral collateral ligament complex. **1 RCL – radial collateral ligament** (arises from the lateral epicondyle and blends with the annular ligament); **2 LUCL – lateral ulnar collateral ligament** (arises posterior to the RCL and attaches to the crista supinatoris of the proximal ulna, just distal to the annular ligament); **3 AL – annular ligament** (attaches to the anterior and posterior margins of the radial notch of the proximal ulna and surrounds the radial head). (**b**) The medial collateral ligament complex. **1 AMCL – anteriomedial collateral ligament** (arises from the antero-inferior medial epicondyle and inserts onto the sublime tubecule of the coronoid process); **2 PMCL – posteromedial collateral ligament** (arises posterior to the AMCL and attaches fan-shaped to the proximal ulna; **3 – Cooper´s ligament** (transverses both bundles)

operative treatment is indicated. Contraindications for a non-operative management are open dislocations, vascular injury and redislocating joints when flexed to less than 30° (Fig. 1.10).

Although the majority of patients will have varus–valgus instability, this fact alone does not automatically indicate surgery. If the patient has the ability to actively stabilize the injured elbow and the muscular origins are diagnosed intact *(→ subchapter symptoms and diagnostics!*), this will be a good qualification for a successful non-operative treatment in author's experience. Consequently, a rehabilitation program including active-assisted and active exercises is essential to maintain concentric reduction while initiating muscle activation. An immediate mobilization does not increase the risk of recurrent instability and leads to improved functional outcomes [38, 39]. However, if the patient is very apprehensive or if the elbow is extremely swollen and painful, a short period of immobilization in a posterior splint may still be indicated. In any case, immobilization longer than 3 weeks should be strictly avoided as this leads to poorer outcomes in elbow range of motion right up to elbow stiffness [5, 38, 40].

In our practice following reduction, the elbow is temporarily immobilized (max. 7 days) in a plaster cast at 90° of elbow flexion with the forearm in pronation, neutral, or supination subject to the direction of main instability. Under physiotherapist's control active-assisted isometric exercises out of the cast are started within the first week. With decreased swelling the cast is replaced by a dynamic brace to mobilize the elbow and to simultaneously minimize shear forces of varus and valgus. The patient is instructed to wear the brace all the time for a total of 6 weeks except when performing exercises. Thereby, the arc of motion is based on the patient's individual degree of stability and apprehension; occasionally an initial extension block (up to 30°) is adjusted according to the reexamined stable arc of motion while the patient is asked to extend and flex the elbow. Moreover, forearm neutral or pronated position can be adjusted to minimize lateral ligamentous stress. Full flexion is usually permitted immediately. Active exercises start from the second week (forearm pronated through the full range of motion; supination with the forearm flexed to 90° or more). Initially, we recommend performing the exercises in an overhead position to ensure maintenance of reduction while utilizing the effects of gravity [41]. Within the first 3 weeks the patient is weekly reexamined. The adjusted extension block should be decreased every week to avoid stiffness in the sequel. Besides, lateral radiographs are performed to confirm joint congruency and to rule out posterolateral subluxation ("drop sign") [42]. After 3–4 weeks the patient should be able to fully extend the elbow and active exercises including forearm rotation are allowed in the sitting/standing position.

After 6 weeks the patient is seen again and the brace is removed. Normal daily activities are resumed and a muscle strengthening is started.

Fig. 1.10 Therapeutic options

Simple elbow dislocation

Non-operative	Operative
Closed dislocation with concentric reduction	Open dislocation
Muscular origins intact– early active ROM possible	Vascular injury
	Redislocation (within functional arc)
	(High demanding patients/ professional athletes)

Sporting activities are not allowed before 3 months after trauma.

Surgical Treatment

A soft tissue exploration and surgical repair is indicated if a closed reduction is not possible or the joint redislocates following closed reduction with a flexion more than 30° (Fig. 1.10) [43]. Based on the current literature surgery is required in less than 10% of patients with simple elbow dislocations treated non-operatively who might develop chronic instability [3, 6]. Nevertheless, especially in high demanding patients like manual labourers or professional athletes the role of surgical management of acute elbow dislocations is still a topic of debate [44]. For these patients a non-surgical treatment with an occasionally required extension block up to 30° (and maybe consequently a prolonged rehabilitation) may not be a suitable option because of their special functional needs. The decision for surgery in these patients therefore depends on the individual's demand and both advantages and drawbacks of surgery should be discussed in detail in every particular case. However at this point, it has to be clearly stated that there is no study to this day showing the superiority of surgical approach over non-operative management [45, 46].

The aim of surgical approach is the concentric joint reduction with direct repair of ligaments and muscle origins. In case of massive ligament disruption the additional augmentation using synthetic tapes (*Internal bracing*) represents a valuable novel option to secure fragile ligament repair and thus to gain primary joint stability. Surgery is performed under general anaesthesia and the instability pattern is clinically reevaluated under muscle relaxation.

Arthroscopy

Prior to open surgical repair an elbow arthroscopy may add the benefit to evaluate joint surfaces, to remove loose bodies (cartilage fragments) and to test/confirm joint stability under direct view (Fig. 1.11a, b) [47]. However, for arthroscopic approach the patient has to be placed in the lateral position that potentially complicates subsequent open soft tissue repair, especially on the medial side. In the author's preferred practice the patient is transferred instead to the supine position following arthroscopy with the affected arm on a radiolucent arm table for soft tissue repair of both sides.

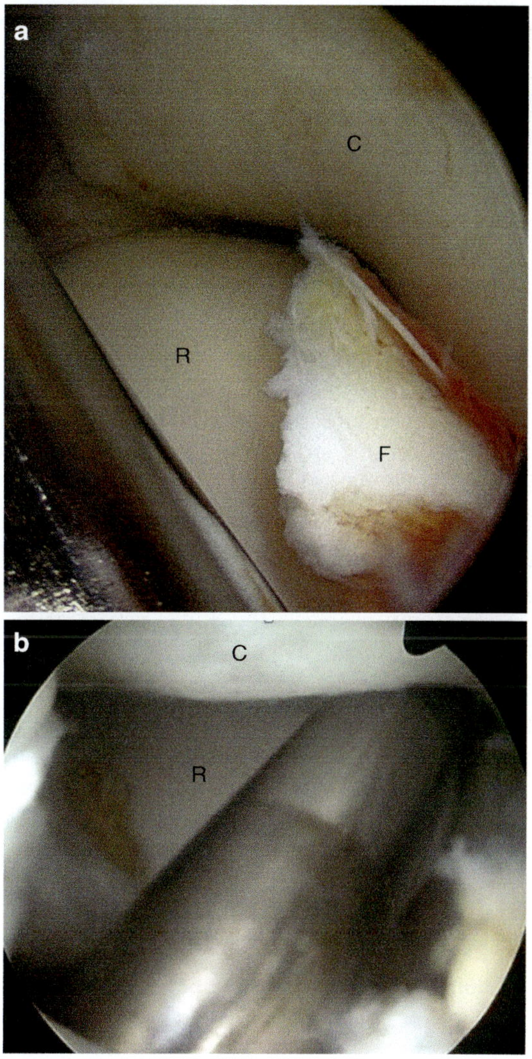

Fig. 1.11 (**a**) View of the antero-lateral joint showing a loose cartilage fragment (F) between the capitelum (C) and the radial head (R) originating from the coroind tip following elbow dislocation. (**b**) View of the postero-lateral joint: the switching stick coming from the soft spot portal "drives through" the radiohumeral joint indicating a posterolateral rotatory instability due to LUCL deficiency (*C* capitellum, *R* radial head)

At this point, it should be noticed that elbow arthroscopy may be significantly complicated in the acute injury due to the disrupted joint capsule resulting in fluid leakage. The arthroscopy following simple elbow dislocation should therefore be reserved for experienced elbow surgeons.

Soft Tissue Repair

Depending on the instability pattern, a lateral, medial or bilateral incision is necessary. In patients with varus or posterolateral rotatory instability the skin incision runs over the lateral epicondyle. In most cases the common extensor mass has been avulsed from the lateral epicondyle together with the LCL complex stripped off the humeral insertion of the capitellum (Fig. 1.12). Typically, a posterior capsular disruption co-occurs and the *Osborne-Cotterill-Lesion* is commonly visible at the dorsal aspect of the capitellum (as the result of the dislocation of the radial head to the back of the capitellum = 'Hill-Sachs-lesion' of the elbow) [48]. Authors prefer to reinsert the ligament complex using a double-loaded suture anchor positioned at the lower margin of the capitellum (center of rotation). Locking stitches are placed into the LCL complex and the extensor fascia as well. Both sutures are then tensioned and knotted with the forearm in 90° of flexion and pronation. Finally, the extensor fascia is additionally stitched and tightened over a drill hole on the lateral epicondyle/supracondylar ridge. For elbows with concomitant MCL instability a medial gapping should be strictly avoided while tensioning the sutures on the lateral side. The congruency of the joint line has to be verified in the a.p.-view via intraoperative fluoroscopy.

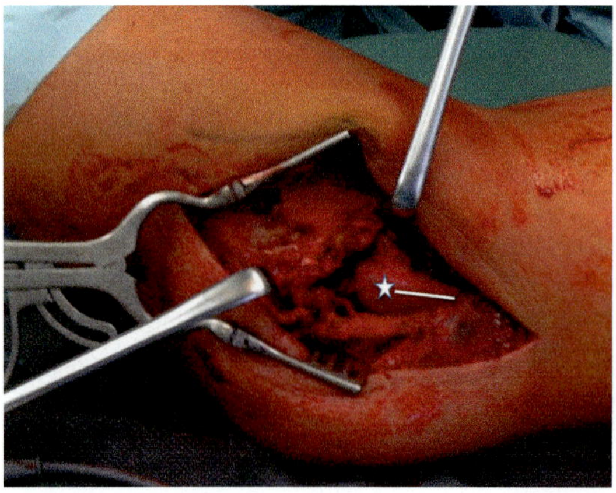

Fig. 1.12 Complete disruption of the common extensor muscles from the lateral epicondyle/supracondylar rigde (star/line)

In case of medial instability or if the elbow remains unstable after LCL repair, the medial side of the elbow is approached via an incision over the medial epicondyle. At first, the ulnar nerve is detected and – if necessary – mobilized for protection throughout the repair procedure. Following skin incision the direct access to the medial aspect of the joint is quite often gained through the massive disrupted flexor-pronator-mass, capsule and MCL complex (Fig. 1.4). Typically, the MCL is avulsed from its humeral insertion. According to the lateral repair, a suture anchor is placed at the center of the arc of the curvature of the trochlea and the MCL as well as the medial capsule are reinserted similary. Last, the flexor-pronator-mass is also repaired with transosseous drill holes.

At the end of the procedure, the joint congruency during range of motion is checked under fluoroscopy again. If the elbow still remains unstable after bilateral soft tissue repair, an external fixation (hinged or static) should be additionally installed.

Internal Bracing

If the disrupted ligament tissue is not suitable for sufficient reinsertion a ligament augmentation (ligament bracing) is useful for repair recruitment. Therefore a synthetic tape is additionally spanned over the sutured ligament complex (Fig. 1.13). In a biomechanical setup, Dugas et al. compared this novel repair technique to medial ligament reconstructions (modified Jobe technique) [49]. They found significantly less gap formation than the reconstruction group and furthermore, there was no difference between groups for maximum torque at failure and torsional stiffness. In the practice of the authors the internal bracing has appeared to be a valuable additional tool to gain primary stability in unstable dislocation injuries. However, to the present day, there is no clinical study reporting results of internal bracing.

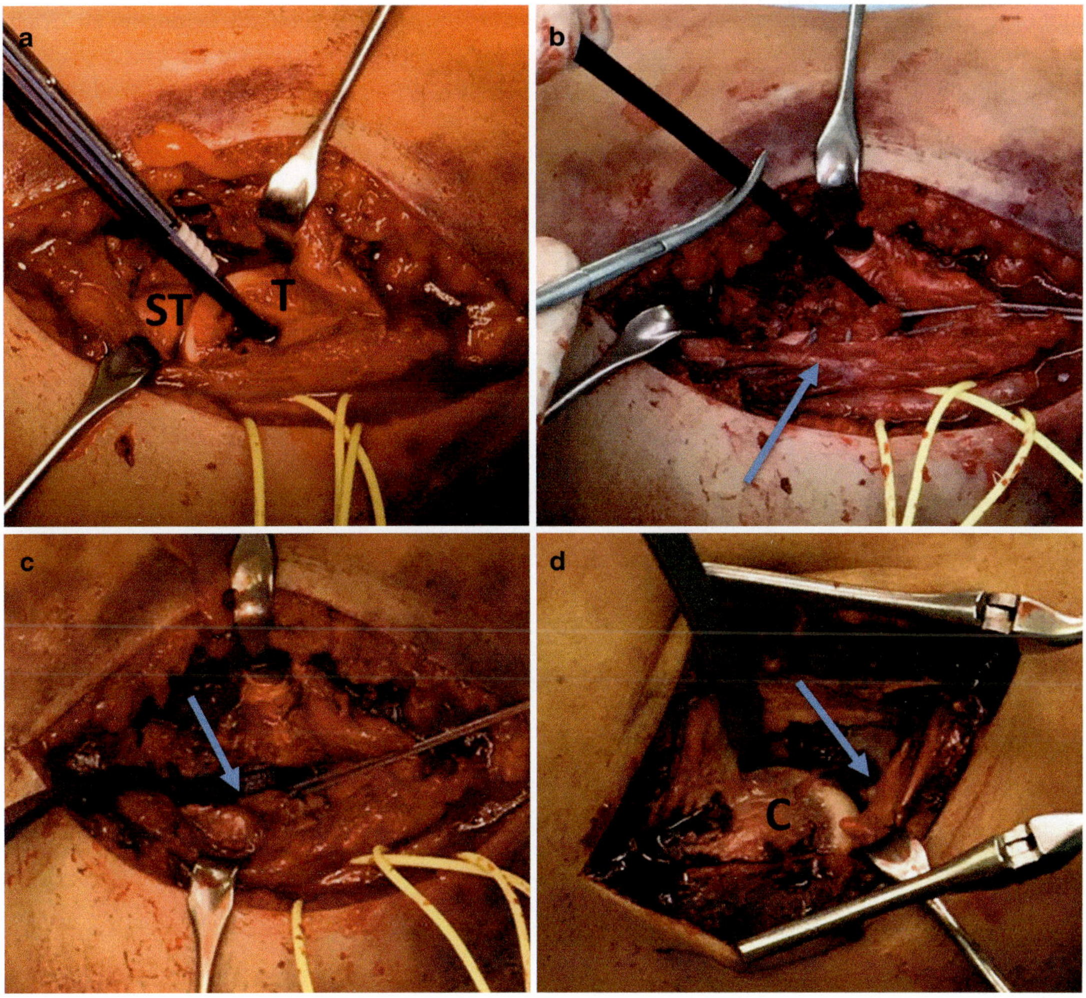

Fig. 1.13 Medial ligament bracing of patient presented in Fig. 1.2: (**a**) Suture anchor implantation additionally loaded with vicryl tape (*ST* sublime tubercule, *T* Trochlea, yellow loops = ulnar nerve); (**b**) following ligament sutering (blue arrow) the tape is spanned back to the sublime tubercule; (**c**) and again fixed with a second bone anchor. (**d**) Also, at the lateral side all soft tissues are stripped off the humerus (*C* capitelum & lateral epicondyle, blue arrow = LUCL)

External Fixation

In the author's approach, an initial external fixation following simple elbow dislocation is reserved for patients with critical soft tissues or obese patients unsuitable for casting/dynamic bracing and soft tissue repair/internal bracing respectively. In these cases a hinged fixator allowing for range of motion exercises (for 4–6 weeks) should be preferred. Also, a static fixator can be used which is more widely available and technically easier to install. According to the non-operative treatment, patients should then be instructed for active excercises utilizing the overhead position after the external fixator is opened by the physical therapist.

Postoperative Care

Following wound closure the elbow is immobilized in a plaster cast at 90° of elbow flexion with the forearm in neutral position. The days following operation passive (CPM – continuous passive motion) and active-assisted isometric excercises start under physiotherapist's control depending on swelling and pain. The postoperative managing protocol is basically guided by the performed ligament repair/bracing and the evaluated elbow stability during surgery as well. In any case a safe arc of motion should be intraoperatively defined – ideally for the full range of motion. To avoid overstretching the repaired ligaments an extension block to 20° is fixed for the first 2 weeks. A dynamic brace is adjusted once swelling has decreased with the appropriate extension block (Fig. 1.14). Especially in patients treated by ligament bracing the CPM and active ROM starting from the first postoperative day to avoid elbow stiffness is crucial.

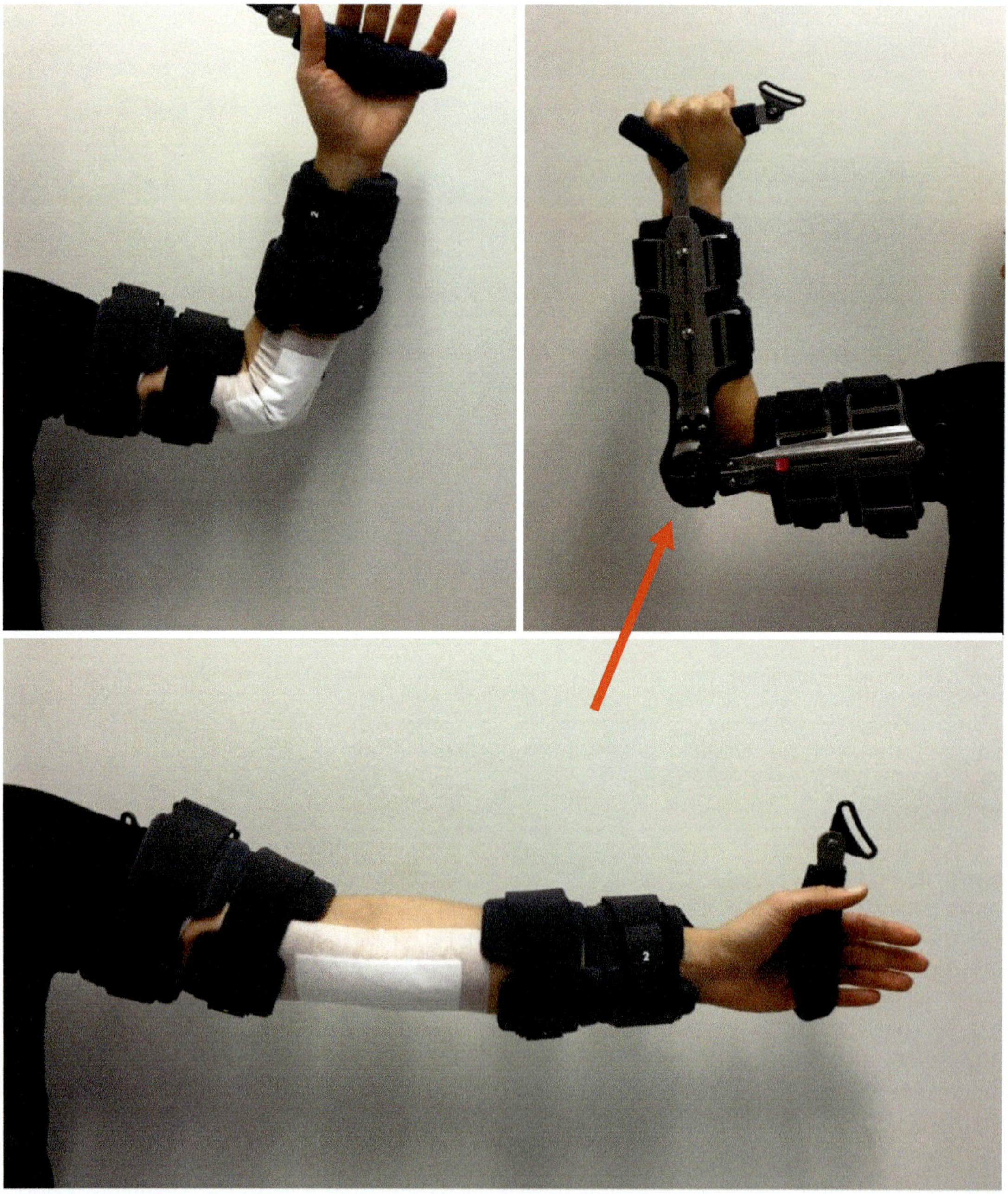

Fig. 1.14 Dynamic brace with adjustable extension block (red arrow)

However, referring to the non-operative treatment active motion should be preferred over passive motion in order to actively center the elbow joint. The overhead position can also be additionally used in the initial rehabilitation period. This position minimizes the effect of gravity, decreases posteriorly directed forces and allows the triceps to function as elbow stabilizer [50]. If both the medial and lateral soft tissue structures have been repaired, active ROM should be initiated with the forearm in neutral position. If the repaired LCL complex has to be protected, the rehabilitation program should be performed with the forearm in pronation. Moreover, shoulder abduction and internal rotation should be strictly avoided to eliminate the gravitational varus, thereby allowing the lateral collateral ligament to heal in an isometric position. To secure the repaired MCL complex and muscle insertion in medially unstable elbows the rehabilitation should conversely be performed in supination. Passive stretching of the elbow is not allowed before the sixth week postoperatively (completion of ligament healing!). Muscle strength training can be started after 6 weeks and sporting activities are allowed after 3 months if joint stability is confirmed.

Outcomes and Complications

For comparing non-operative and surgical treatment Josefsson and colleagues carried out two studies [45, 46]. Both studies show no significant differences in treatment of ligamentous injuries after simple elbow dislocation. However, both studies did not differentiate the severity of soft tissue injuries in evaluated patients. In a current survey, the importance of the extent of soft tissue injury is highlighted, based on patients' results requiring surgery due to recurrent instability after non-operative treatment [6]. In addition to this, surgical implants and techniques have improved tremendously over the last decades allowing less invasive approaches and early functional rehabilitation programs.

Although the long-term results of conservative treatment are considered good to excellent in most patients, an increased risk of degenerative changes causing elbow pain is verified [51]. Residual instability and/or restrictions in elbow movement (joint contractures) are also reported in the sequel of non-operative treatment. Motion deficits and elbow stiffness are distinctly correlated to an immobilization longer than 2–3 weeks [38–40, 52].

For primary ligament repair good functional results are reported via open or arthroscopic approach in the short-to midterm follow-up [7, 53–58]. Kim et al. showed better MEPI scores for patients with unilateral versus bilateral ligament reconstruction [54]. Due to inadequate diagnostics, misjudgement of injury severity or failed/insufficient repair however, subluxation may persist leading to elbow pain and/or stiffness in some circumstances following surgery. The prompt detection of the complete injury extent is crucial to initiate adequate treatment. Otherwise, a delayed treatment quite often necessitates LCL and MCL reconstruction using autologuos graft ligaments following extensive elbow arthrolysis [23, 47, 55]. Nevertheless, Daluski et al. reported no differences in clinical outcome or range of motion after direct ligament repair without supplemental tendon graft reconstruction of the LUCL between acute (<30 days) and delayed (>30 days) treated patients [56].

To prevent elbow stiffness after surgical repair, early postoperative (active) motion is mandatory. While recurrent instability is reported in rare cases, some patients may require elbow release or excision of heterotopic bone to regain full range of motion. As mentioned before, no data exist for internal bracing in the current literature. The benefits/drawbacks and possible complications of this novel technique have to be reviewed in the future.

References

1. Stoneback JW, Owens BD, Sykes J, Athwal GS, Pointer L, Wolf JM. Incidence of elbow dislocations in the United States population. J Bone Joint Surg Am. 2012;94:240–5.
2. Josefsson PO, Johnell O, Gentz CF. Long-term sequelae of simple dislocation of the elbow. J Bone Joint Surg Am. 1984;66:927–30.
3. Anakwe RE, Middleton SD, Jenkins PJ, McQueen MM, Court-Brown CM. Patient-reported outcomes after simple dislocation of the elbow. J Bone Joint Surg Am. 2011;93:1220–6.

4. Josefsson PO, Nilsson BE. Incidence of elbow dislocation. Acta Orthop Scand. 1986;57:537–8.
5. Mehlhoff TL, Noble PC, Bennett JB, Tullos HS. Simple dislocation of the elbow in the adult. Results after closed treatment. J Bone Joint Surg Am. 1988;70:244–9.
6. Modi CS, Wasserstein D, Mayne IP, Henry PD, Mahomed N, Veillette CJ. The frequency and risk factors for subsequent surgery after a simple elbow dislocation. Injury. 2015;46:1156–60.
7. Duckworth AD, Ring D, Kulijdian A, et al. Unstable elbow dislocations. J Shoulder Elbow Surg. 2008;17(2):281–6.
8. Hackl M, Beyer F, Wegmann K, Leschinger T, Burkhart KJ, Müller LP. The treatment of simple elbow dislocation in adults. Dtsch Arztebl Int. 2015;112(18):311–9.
9. Rotini R. An overview about elbow instability. Musculoskelet Surg. 2014;98(Suppl 1):S1–3.
10. Marinelli A, Guerra A, Rotini R. Elbow instability: are we able to classify it? Review of the literature and proposal of an all-inclusive classification system. Musculoskelet Surg. 2016;100(Suppl 1):S61–71.
11. Hildebrand KA, Patterson SD, King GJ. Acute elbow dislocations: simple and complex. Orthop Clin North Am. 1999;30(1):63–79.
12. Morrey BF. Acute and chronic instability of the elbow. J Am Acad Orthop Surg. 1996;4:117–28.
13. Ring D, Jupiter J. Fracture-dislocation of the elbow. J Bone J Surg Am. 1998;4:566–80.
14. Chan K, King GJW, Faber KJ. Treatment of complex elbow fracture-dislocations. Curr Rev Musculoskelet Med. 2016;9(2):185–9.
15. O'Driscoll SW. Classification and evaluation of recurrent instability of the elbow. Clin Orthop Relat Res. 2000;370:34–43.
16. Siebenlist S, Reeps C, Kraus T, Martetschläger F, Schmitt A, Stöckle U, Freude T. Brachial artery transection caused by closed elbow dislocation in a mature in-line skater: a case report with review of the literature. Knee Surg Sports Traumatol Arthrosc. 2010;18(12):1667–70.
17. Biberthaler P, Kanz KG, Siebenlist S. Elbow joint dislocation - important considerations for closed reduction. MMW Fortschr Med. 2015;157(9):50–2.
18. Pipicelli JG, Chinchalkar SJ, Grewal R, King GJ. Therapeutic implications of the radiographic "drop sign" following elbow dislocation. J Hand Ther. 2012;25(3):346–53.
19. Hackl M, Wegmann K, Ries C, Leschinger T, Burkhart KJ, Müller LP. Reliability of magnetic resonance imaging signs of posterolateral rotatory instability of the elbow. J Hand Surg Am. 2015;40(7):1428–33.
20. Schnetzke M, Aytac S, Studier-Fischer S, Grützner PA, Guehring T. Initial joint stability affects the outcome after conservative treatment of simple elbow dislocations: a retrospective study. J Orthop Surg Res. 2015;10:128.
21. Robinson PM, Griffiths E, Watts AC. Simple elbow dislocation. Shoulder Elbow. 2017;9(3):195–204.
22. Adolfsson LE, Nestorson JO, Scheer JH. Extensive soft tissue lesions in redislocated after simple elbow dislocations. J Shoulder Elbow Surg. 2017;26(7):1294–7.
23. O'Driscoll SW, Bell DF, Morrey BF. Posterolateral rotatory instability of the elbow. J Bone Joint Surg Am. 1991;73:440–6.
24. O'Driscoll SW, Morrey BF, Korinek S, An KN. Elbow subluxation and dislocation. A spectrum of instability. Clin Orthop Relat Res. 1992;280:186–97.
25. Schwab GH, Bennett JB, Woods GW, Tullos HS. Biomechanics of elbow instability: the role of the medial collateral ligament. Clin Orthop Relat Res. 1980;146:42–52.
26. Søjbjerg JO, Helmig P, Kjaersgaard-Andersen P. Dislocation of the elbow: an experimental study of the ligamentous injuries. Orthopedics. 1989;12:461–3.
27. Rhyou IH, Kim YS. New mechanism of the posterior elbow dislocation. Knee Surg Sports Traumatol Arthrosc. 2012;20:2535–41.
28. Schreiber JJ, Warren RF, Hotchkiss RN, Daluiski A. An online video investigation into the mechanism of elbow dislocation. J Hand Surg Am. 2013;38:488–94.
29. Schreiber JJ, Potter HG, Warren RF, Hotchkiss RN, Daluiski A. Magnetic resonance imaging findings in acute elbow dislocation: insight into mechanism. J Hand Surg Am. 2014;39:199–205.
30. Morrey BF, An KN. Articular and ligamentous contributions to the stability of the elbow joint. Am J Sports Med. 1983;11:315–9.
31. Olsen BS, Søjbjerg JO, Dalstra M, Sneppen O. Kinematics of the lateral ligamentous constraints of the elbow joint. J Shoulder Elbow Surg. 1996;5:333–41.
32. Callaway GH, Field LD, Deng XH, et al. Biomechanical evaluation of the medial collateral ligament of the elbow. J Bone Joint Surg Am. 1997;79:1223–31.
33. Safran MR, Baillargeon D. Soft-tissue stabilizers of the elbow. J Shoulder Elbow Surg. 2005;14(1 Suppl S):179–85.
34. Pereira BP. Revisiting the anatomy and biomechanics of the anconeus muscle and its role in elbow stability. Ann Anat. 2013;195:365–70.
35. Dunning CE, Zarzour ZD, Patterson SD, Johnson JA, King GJ. Muscle forces and pronation stabilize the lateral ligament deficient elbow. Clin Orthop Relat Res. 2001;388:118–24.
36. Armstrong AD, Dunning CE, Faber KJ, Duck TR, Johnson JA, King GJ. Rehabilitation of the medial collateral ligament-deficient elbow: an in vitro biomechanical study. J Hand Surg Am. 2000;25:1051–7.
37. Seiber K, Gupta R, McGarry MH, Safran MR, Lee TQ. The role of the elbow musculature, forearm rotation, and elbow flexion in elbow stability: an in vitro study. J Shoulder Elbow Surg. 2009;18:260–8.
38. Maripuri SN, Debnath UK, Rao P, Mohanty K. Simple elbow dislocation among adults: a comparative study of two different methods of treatment. Injury. 2007;38:1254–8.

39. Lordens GI, Van Lieshout EM, Schep NW, et al. Early mobilisation versus plaster immobilisation of simple elbow dislocations: results of the FuncSiE multicentre randomised clinical trial. Br J Sports Med. 2015; https://doi.org/10.1136/bjsports-2015-094704.
40. Panteli M, Pountos I, Kanakaris NK, Tosounidis TH, Giannoudis PV. Cost analysis and outcomes of simple elbow dislocations. World J Orthop. 2015;6:513–20.
41. Schreiber JJ, Paul S, Hotchkiss RN, Daluiski A. Conservative management of elbow dislocations with an overhead motion protocol. J Hand Surg Am. 2015;40(3):515–9.
42. Coonrad RW, Roush TF, Major NM, Basamania CJ. The drop sign, a radiographic warning sign of elbow instability. J Shoulder Elbow Surg. 2005;14:312–7.
43. O'Driscoll SW, Jupiter JB, King GJ, Hotchkiss RN, Morrey BF. The unstable elbow. Instr Course Lect. 2001;50:89–102.
44. Savoie FH III, Trenhaile SW, Roberts J, Field LD, Ramsey JR. Primary repair of ulnar collateral ligament injuries of the elbow in young athletes: a case series of injuries to the proximal and distal ends of the ligament. Am J Sports Med. 2008;36:1066–10672.
45. Josefsson PO, Gentz CF, Johnell O, Wendeberg B. Surgical versus non-surgical treatment of ligamentous injuries following dislocation of the elbow joint. A prospective randomized study. J Bone Joint Surg Am. 1987;69:605–8.
46. Josefsson PO, Gentz CF, Johnell O, Wendeberg B. Surgical versus nonsurgical treatment of ligamentous injuries following dislocations of the elbow joint. Clin Orthop Relat Res. 1987;214:165–9.
47. Savoie FH III, O'Brien MJ, Field LD, Gurley DJ. Arthroscopic and open radial ulnohumeral ligament reconstruction for posterolateral rotatory instability of the elbow. Clin Sports Med. 2010;29:611–8.
48. Osborne G, Cotterill P. Recurrent dislocation of the elbow. J Bone Joint Surg Br. 1966;48(2):340–6.
49. Dugas JR, Walters BL, Beason DP, Fleisig GS, Chronister JE. Biomechanical comparison of ulnar collateral ligament repair with internal bracing versus modified Jobe reconstruction. Am J Sports Med. 2016;44:735–41.
50. Manocha RH, Kusins JR, Johnson JA, King GJ. Optimizing the rehabilitation of elbow lateral collateral ligament injuries: a biomechanical study. J Shoulder Elbow Surg. 2016;26(4):596–603.
51. Eygendaal D, Verdegaal SH, Obermann WR, et al. Posterolateral dislocation of the elbow joint. Relationship to medial instability. J Bone Joint Surg Am. 2000;82:555–60.
52. Rafai M, Largab A, Cohen D, Trafeh M. Pure posterior luxation of the elbow in adults: immobilization or early mobilization. A randomized prospective study of 50 cases. Chir Main. 1999;18:272–8.
53. Jeon IH, Kim SY, Kim PT. Primary ligament repair for elbow dislocation. Keio J Med. 2008;57:99–104.
54. Kim BS, Park KH, Song HS, Park SY. Ligamentous repair of acute lateral collateral ligament rupture of the elbow. J Shoulder Elbow Surg. 2013;22:1469–73.
55. Sanchez-Sotelo J, Morrey BF, O'Driscoll SW. Ligamentous repair and reconstruction for posterolateral rotatory instability of the elbow. J Bone Joint Surg Br. 2005;87:54–61.
56. Daluiski A, Schrumpf MA, Schreiber JJ, Nguyen JT, Hotchkiss RN. Direct repair for managing acute and chronic lateral ulnar collateral ligament disruptions. J Hand Surg Am. 2014;39:1125–9.
57. O'Brien MJ, Savoie FH 3rd. Arthroscopic and open management of posterolateral rotatory instability of the elbow. Sports Med Arthrosc. 2014;22:194–200.
58. O'Brien MJ, Lee Murphy R, Savoie FH 3rd. A preliminary report of acute and subacute arthroscopic repair of the radial ulnohumeral ligament after elbow dislocation in the high-demand patient. Arthroscopy. 2014;30:679–87.

Traumatic Rotatory Instability of the Elbow

2

Posterolateral Rotatory Instability (PLRI) and Posteromedial Rotatory Instability (PMRI)

Andreas Lenich, Sebastian Siebenlist, and Andreas B. Imhoff

Epidemiology

The epidemiology of elbow rotatory instability is until now not fully understood. The phenomen of various elbow instabilities as the posterolateral rotatory instability (PLRI) is multiple described but the pathomechanism for a posterior medial rotatory instability (PMRI) could not be simulated until now. Especially the combined injuries of the fracture of a coronoid and ligament ruptures could not be identified by the classification of Regan and Morrey [1]. The PMRI was first described by O'Driscoll et al. [2] in 2003 as anteromedial fractures of the coronoid (AMC) and lateral varus instability. After acute trauma these fractures are often missed because of their rarity. Moreover, associated to coronoid fractures they often look subtle like terrible triad injuries. This might lead to poor clinical outcomes. Further teaching in diagnostics, understanding of the rotatory pathomechanism and treatment has to be trained to reduce the rate of insuffizient outcome of the PMRI and PLRI, respectively.

Pathomechanism

As the elbow is such a stable construct for a rotatory instability severe valgus (PMRI) or varus (PLRI) load is needed. The mechanism of posterolateral rotatory elbow instability is described in detail in chapter "Simple elbow dislocations".

In case of a valgus overload the radial collateral ligament will rupture and on the other side a concave fracture in the anterior coronoid can be seen. This leads to a PMRI. G. King described the pathomechanism for the anteromedial coronoid fracture (O'Driscoll Type II) occuring by pronation, varus, and axially directed forces [3]. It is accompanied by avulsion injuries of the LCL and the posterior bundle of the MCL. Injury to the anterior bundle of the MCL can also occur with anterior medial coronoid (AMC) fractures and will enhance the elbow instability [2, 3].

In case of a varus overload the lateral ulnar collateral ligament will rupture and in some elbows a convex fracture of the anterior coronoid rim can be seen. If seen in chronic cases the ROM might be reduced or the picture of a stiff joint can be found.

A. Lenich (✉)
Department of Trauma- and Sportorthopaedic Surgery, Helios Klinikum München West, Munich, Germany

S. Siebenlist · A. B. Imhoff
Department of Orthopaedic Sports Medicine, Technical University Munich Klinikum rechts der Isar, Munich, Germany
e-mail: sebastian.siebenlist@tum.de; imhoff@tum.de

P. Biberthaler et al. (eds.), *Acute Elbow Trauma*, Strategies in Fracture Treatments,
https://doi.org/10.1007/978-3-319-97850-5_2

Clinical Signs

In acute trauma the patients have a free range of motion with an instability feeling when testing them with light varus or valgus resistance. There might be haematoma medial and lateral at the joint. Sensomotoric deficits are very seldom but have to e securly excluded. In chronic cases, patients often describe persistent pain and cannot remember any previous trauma.

Because of the short history of realization and published AMC fractures the incidence of associated injuries is not well known. The partial or complete injuries of the LCL are common and the amount of injuries to the posterior bundle of the MCL is uncertain. As well known in terrible triad injuries there is a fracture of the radial head but not in patients with anteromedial coronoid fractures and a consecutive PMRI. So this is a fact to differentiate and to detect the PMRI.

As published by G. King the PMRI should be suspected in any patient who appears to have an anteromedial coronoid fracture when a radial head fracture is not present [3, 4].

The following clinical examination should be verified in the case of suspected elbow instability:

The PLRI testings:

- Valgus stress Test (intensifier in 0–30–60°)
- Drawer Test
- Pivot shift Test
- Pincer grip Test
- Push up Test

The PMRI testings:

- Varus stress test
- Arm lift up test (Intensifier)

Associated Injuries

The associated injuries are depending on the severity of trauma. The isolated ligament rupture (especially LCL) up to an terrible triad injury (see also chapter "Terrible triad") can be found. The frequency of an injury to the posterior bundle of the MCL is not well documented. In varus/valgus injuries with rotational instability even the wrist has to be investigated to detect further possible instabilities.

Classification

PMRI Classification (Coronoid Fracture Classification)

In the publication of O'Driscoll et al. [2] three anteromedial coronoid fracture subtypes are differentiated. Subtype I involves the anteromedial rim only, subtype II involves the rim and tip with an concave fracture line, and subtype III involves the rim, and sublime tubercle, with or without involvement of the tip. (Fig. 2.1).

PLRI Classification

The PLRI can be classified after O'Driscoll according to the grade of the joint dislocation [5, 6] between 0 and 3. No statement can be given about the clinical instability. Geyer et al. published an arthroscopy based classification [7]. Because every ligament can be seperatly tested, this gives a highly differenciated diagnose.

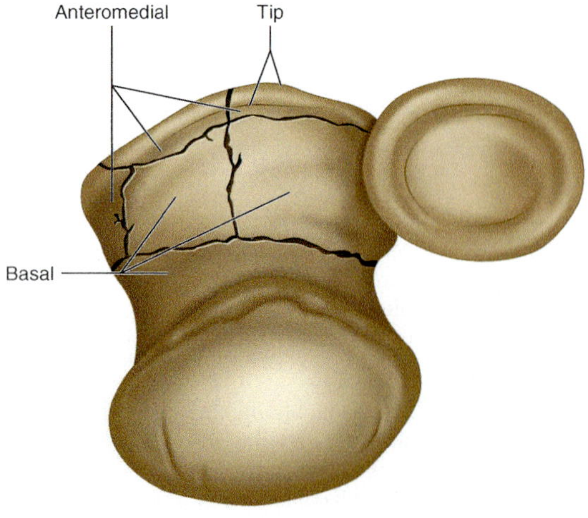

Fig. 2.1 Coronoid fracture classification after O'Driscoll

Symptoms and Diagnostics

Signs and Symptoms of Posteromedial Rotatory Instability of the Elbow (PMRI)

Every injured or dislocated elbow has to be examinated in detail about neurovascular injury before and after reduction. The status of soft tissue and the condition of the skin should be carefully assessed and documented. Also a carefully palpation for signs of tenderness, particularly over the LCL, MUCL and LUCL is recommended. If a patient complains of crepitus within elbow motion, the arm in valgus stress abducted from the side, this might be cartilage crepitus due to maltracking in varus PMRI [8, 9].

Signs and Symptoms of Posterolateral Rotatory Instability of the Elbow (PLRI)

Beside the mentioned common examinations in injured elbows the PLRI shows specific symtoms in clinical examination tests like the pivot shift stress test, the drawer test, the push up test and the relocation test of the elbow. In the acute phase the patient reports an instability and weekness in elbow valgus stress situations. In the chronic phase some patients show the symptoms of a radial epicondylopathy and in a later phase a neuritis of the ulnar nerve can be seen.

Rotatory Instability: Imaging

In the acute trauma X-ray in AP, lateral views (Fig. 2.2) and if there is a painful region around the radial head a targeting picture or the radial head is recommended. If clinically indicated X-rays of the shoulder, forearm, and wrist can be made. After the reduction of an elbow dislocation the standard X-rays of the elbow has to be repeated. Findings can be subtle, such as loss of a parallel medial ulnohumeral joint line, or varus malalignment of the elbow [10]. The radiocapitellar joint may be widened with LCL disruption and a "fake" fragment from the lateral condyle may be visible. CT scans (Fig. 2.3) with 3-D reconstruction (Fig. 2.4) improve the recognition and understanding of the pattern of anteromedial coronoid fractures are recommended routinely in the evaluation of these injuries [11].

The use of the MRI in these cases is still under discussion. In acute trauma if prompt available the extra information about muscle leasions can give the treatment indication. In chronic cases the stress test under ultrasound vision is also recommendable.

Injury Pattern and Surgery Related Anatomy

The combination of LCL injury and an anteromedial coronoid fracture showed in biomechanical test a fragment size depending

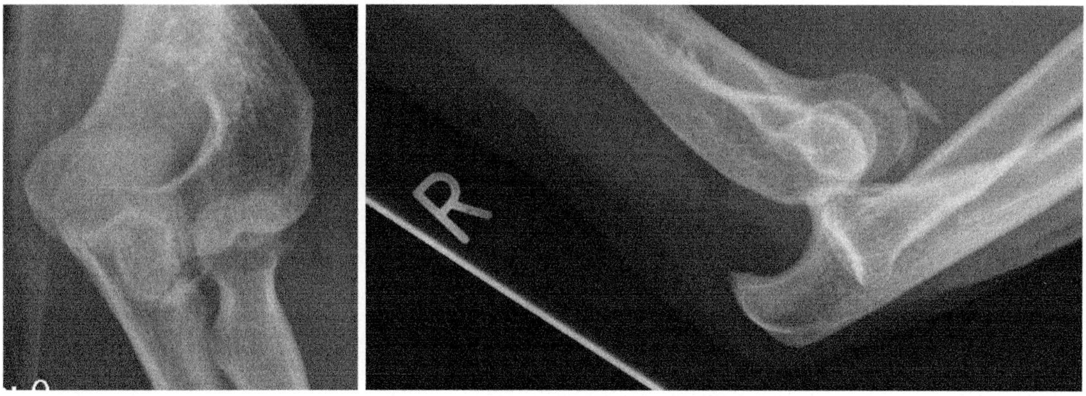

Fig. 2.2 A.P. and lateral view of the dislocated right elbow joint with coronoid fragments in front of the trochlea humeri

instability. G.King recommends the internal fixation of the lateral Ligament and the coronoid fragment if larger than 2.5 mm [12]. However, we have seen severe complications in patients with only ligament repair and we therefore recommend also to reconstruct or to buttress small coronoid fractures to give the elbow more varus stability.

The stability of the sublime tubercule has also to be controlled. Discontinuity of the sublime tubercule is often combined with MCL instability and has to be surgically addressed.

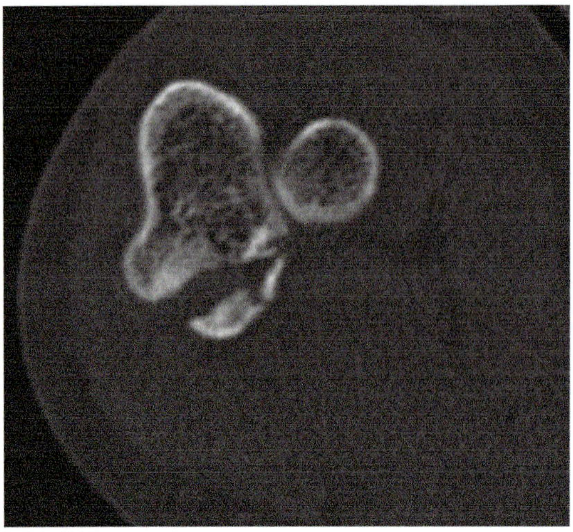

Fig. 2.3 Coronar CT Scan view of the coronoid and medial facet with a concave fragment of the medial coronoid

Therapeutic Options

Non-operative Treatment

The conservative treatment of PMRI and PLRI dependes of several factors. In the international literature there is no clear recommendation for or against. If there is no contious dislocation of the elbow, the coronoid fragment is small and the patient is compliant a non operative treatment can be initiated. An ultrasound or intensifyer examination can clear the indication. Large coronoid fragments, additional muscle injury, continous subluxation or dislocation require operative treatment. Sometimes a CT scan showes a joint incongruacy not seen in the X-ray.

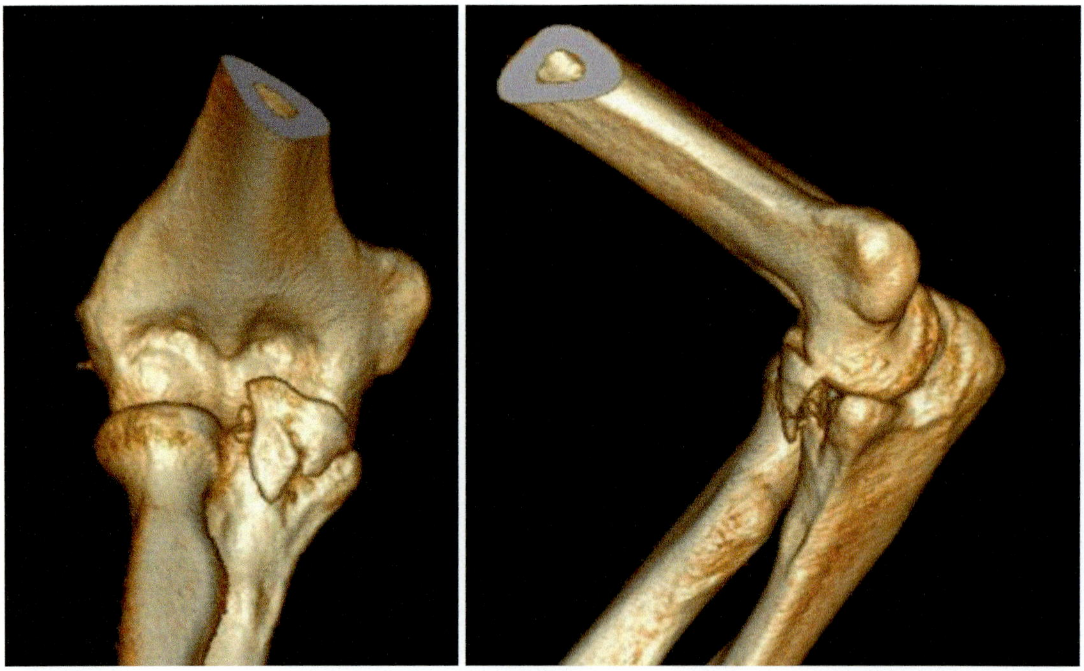

Fig. 2.4 3D reconstructed CT Scan with a coronoid fragment Type II after the O'Driscoll classification

Anteromedial Coronoid Fracture

The non-operative treatment of anteromedial coronoid fractures starts with a cast in 90° elbow flexion with the forearm in neutral rotation for 1 week. Passiv motion out of the cast once a day with the help of a physiotherapist is recommended from the beginning. After 1 week the patient gets an orthesis for the daytime with a limitation in the individual stable arc. The patient should aktively start with extension and flexion without weight-bearing for minimum of 6 weeks. The cast is still a good option during the night. Passive motion out of the stable arc should be done by the phyiotherapist. If crepitus occures the diagnostic has to be focused and a surgical treatment might be needed.

Because of a varus moment on the elbow the abduction of the arm should be avoided.

Further we read in the book of G. King that, pronation stabilizes the LCL de cient elbow, supination stabilizes the coronoid de cient elbow; hence neutral rotation is selected for flexion and extension exercises and for immobilization.

We recommend weekly clinical and X-ray control to monitor fracture displacement and ROM. A reduction of the ROM and/or a subluxation/dislocation is an indication for an operation. The Patient shouldn't practice with load until the full range of motion or the 12 week isn't reached.

In the literature the information regarding outcome of nonoperative PMRI of the elbow is low. Doornberg and King reported on 18 patients with anteromedial facet fractures with an average follow-up of 26 months. Three patients had nonoperative treatment, and two had an excellent outcome and one fair [13].

Because a fragment malunion may lead to persistent subluxation and secondary osteoarthritis for which there is currently no good reconstructive option we prefere inthe most of the cases the surgical treatment.

Surgical Treatment PMRI

The indication for surgical treatment is given in Patients with nonconcentric elbow, displaced anteromedial coronoid fracture, fracture fragment interposed in elbow articulation.

Under anaestehsia the elbow stability can be tested under an intensifierto proof the colateral ligament instability and fragment dislocation under load.

For the patient positioning an arm table can be used. The posteromedial rotatory instability injuries of the elbow are best approached with a medial incision. Herefore a high shoulder rotation of more than 90° is needed. As an alternative the injury can be repaired with the arm placed across the chest.

For the preoperative planning a CT scan is helpfull for fragment size and number. The main fragments like the medial facett and large anterior coronoid tip fragments has to be adressed with a stabel osteosynthesis. We recomend to use 2.4 mm interlocking plates and screws for radial head and coronoid. After the osteosynthesis, ruptured ligaments (LCL) has to be fixed by suture anchors, in our hands 2.5–3.5 mm diameter. If the sublime tubercule is fractured we also fix it with suture anchors. 1.6 and 2.0 mm K-wires are also needed.

The surgical approach to the coronoid fracture is described as anterior or medial (Fig. 2.5). If only the ulnar side hast o be done, we prefer in the acute traumatic situation the medial access. To reach the LCL and the radial head the Kochers approach is recomended.

The ulnar nerv has to be located safely. If preoperative ulnaris nerve symptomes are documented a decompression of the nerv and if needed a ventral transposition should be done. We also recommend to do a transposition oft he nerve in cases of medial ulnar plate osteosynthesis.

The best approach to reach the anteromedial coronoid fractures is the interval between the heads of the flexor carpi ulnaris muscle. By using this approach the sublime tubercule and the MCL can also be reconstructed.

For the reconstruction of the coronoid tip (Subtype II fracture) the flexor pronator muscle has to be detached from the medial epicondyle plus the supracondylar ridge. A temporary fixation with K wires allowes the final osteosynthesis with canulated screws or or interlocking plates after a controll of the position with the intensifier. Because a rigide fixation is needed for the coronoid fractures a suture fixation is not recommended. (Fig. 2.6).

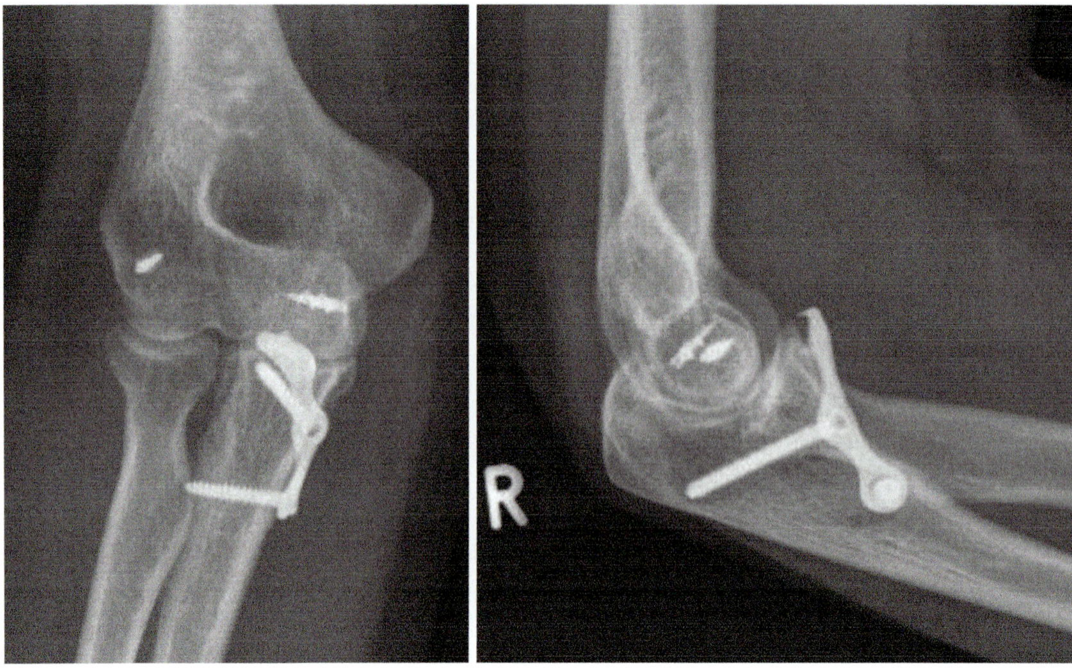

Fig. 2.5 Medial approach to the Elbow joint and the coronoid tip

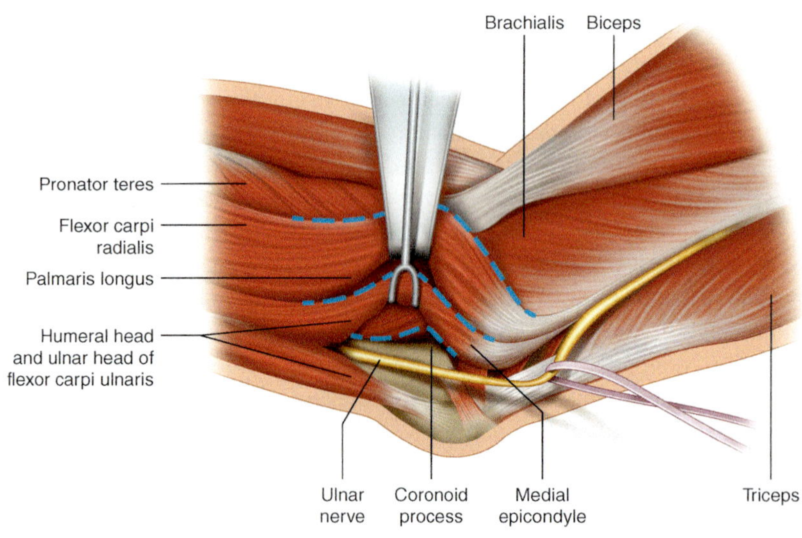

Fig. 2.6 Postoperative elbow X-rays in a.p. and lateral view after osteosynthesis with an interlocking plate for the coronoid Type II fragment and two suture anchors to fix the flexor tendon on the medial epicondyle and the LUCL on the lateral side

In the next step the LCL stability is tested with the intensifier under a mild valgus stress. If the joint gap opens up wide (more than double) a reconstruction will be done over the Kochers approach (Fig. 2.7) and the ligaments can be fixed with suture anchors. (Fig. 2.6).

The stability will now be tested in mild valgus and varus stress test under an intensifier. If there is an residual instability a fixateur externe can be used.

Surgical Treatment PLRI

In acute trauma in the PLRI cases there might be seen a rupture of the LCL and LUCL. Sometimes a konvex fragment of the medial coronoid can be found. This is biomechanicaly discussed as a pushed out fragment. The Kochers aproach and a split between the extensor carpi brevis and the

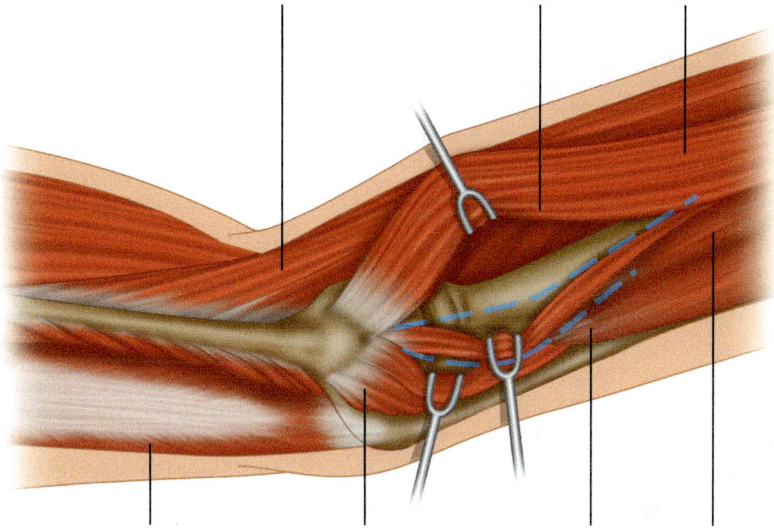

Fig. 2.7 Lateral approach to the Elbow joint with the possibility of Kochers and Kaplan approaches

anconeus muscle gives a good visualisation on the subepicondyle region. If possible the ligaments can be reconstructed by a base ball stich and a suture anchor in the isometric region of the lateral epicondyle (Fig. 2.6).

If a coronoid fragment is present it either has to be removed or fixed to prevent medial instability. The instability can be tested with mild varus stress under the intensifier.

The operation technique is similar to the PMRI treatment.

Postoperative Care

In the OR the Elbow is placed in a 90° splint with imobilisation of the wrist in intrinsic plus position. On the first postoperative day the passiv mobilisation out of the cast by the physiotherapist beginns. The cast has to be woren for a minimum of 5 days. After that a moving orthesis can be used for 6 weeks. We recommend to use the orthese by day and the cast by night untill the first 14 postop days for faster reduction of the oedema. First 2 weeks ROM in extension/flexion 0–20–90° and no pro- or supination, 3–4 week ROM in extension/flexion 0–10–110° and free pro- or supination, 5–6 week in extension/flexion 0-0-free and free pro- or supination. After the 6th week physikal examination with load is allowed.

Outcomes and Complications

After stable fixation of the cornoid fragments complications are rare. Non rigide stabilisation leads to subluxation and destruction of the elbow joint.

The ulnaris nerve reacts sometimes sensible to contact with plates or screws. Thats why in these cases a transposition is recommended.

There is a limited number of case reports in the literature about PLRI and PMRI injuries and treatment. Doornberg and Ring published a retrospective review about 67 elbow dislocations with 11 patients having a varus posteromedial instability [14]. Another study of these authors presented 18 patients with anteromedial facet fractures of the coronoid and in 12 cases exelent results after stable anatomical fixation of the fragments [13].

Conclusion

PMRI and PLRI are rare injuries and have not to be missed. Surgical treatment seems to be a good option for exellent results if a stable anatomical fixation is reached.

References

1. Regan W, Morrey B. Fractures of the coronoid process of the ulna. J Bone Joint Surg Am. 1989;71(9):1348–54.
2. O'Driscoll SW, Jupiter JB, Cohen MS, et al. Difficult elbow fractures: pearls and pitfalls. Instr Course Lect. 2003;52:113–34.
3. Beingessner DM, Whitcomb Pollock J, King GJW. Introduction to posteromedial rotatory instability (PMRI) of the elbow 1304-Rockwood. 2014, Chapter 12.
4. Ring D, Jupiter JB, Zilberfarb J. Posterior dislocation of the elbow with fractures of the radial head and coronoid. J Bone Joint Surg Am. 2002;84A(4):547–51.
5. O'Driscoll SW, Morrey BF, Korinek S, et al. Elbow subluxation and dislocation. A spectrum of instability. Clin Orthop. 1992;280:186–97.
6. Dunning CE, Zarzour ZD, Patterson SD, et al. Muscle forces and pronation stabilize the lateral ligament deficient elbow. Clin Orthop. 2001;388:118–24.
7. Geyer M, Schoch C, Harnoß T. Therapiemöglichkeiten der chronischen ligamentären Ellenbogeninstabilität. Arthroskopie. 2013;26:197–206.
8. Sanchez-Sotelo J, O'Driscoll SW, Morrey BF. Medial oblique compression fracture of the coronoid process of the ulna. J Shoulder Elbow Surg. 2005;14(1):60–4.
9. Ring D. Fractures of the coronoid process of the ulna. J Hand Surg Am. 2006;31(10):1679–89.
10. Taylor TK, Scham SM. A posteromedial approach to the proximal end of the ulna for the internal fixation of olecranon fractures. J Trauma. 1969;9(7):594–602.
11. Lindenhovius A, Karanicolas PJ, Bhandari M, et al. Interobserver reliability of coronoid fracture classification: two-dimensional versus three-dimensional computed tomography. J Hand Surg Am. 2009;34(9):1640–6.
12. Pollock JW, Brownhill J, Ferreira L, et al. The effect of anteromedial facet fractures of the coronoid and lateral collateral ligament injury on elbow stability and kinematics. J Bone Joint Surg Am. 2009;91(6):1448–58.
13. Doornberg JN, Ring DC. Fracture of the anteromedial facet of the coronoid process. J Bone Joint Surg Am. 2006;88(10):2216–24.
14. Doornberg JN, Ring D. Coronoid fracture patterns. J Hand Surg Am. 2006;31(1):45–52.

Distal Humerus Fractures

3

Arne Berner, Michael Leopold Nerlich, Ulrich Stöckle, and Markus A. E. Gühring

Epidemiology

Fractures of the distal humerus are rare but severe injuries with an estimated incidence in adults of 5.7 per 100,000 persons per year, only a small proportion of 2–3% of the population of all fractures are related to the distal humerus [1]. In most of the cases these fractures are treated surgically to ensure good functional outcome of the elbow. In younger people more man are involved and they are mostly associated with high energy trauma. In elderly people the fractures are caused by low-energy trauma. A predominance in women is mostly found in combination with osteoporotic bone quality, which makes the operative treatment more challenging. In a recent study Palvanen et al. reported an increase in the annual incidence of distal humeral fractures in older women (over 60 years of age) from twelve per 100,000 to thirty-four per 100,000 during the time from 1970 to 1998 [2].

Based on the increasing number of fractures in the elderly treatment strategies have to consider fixation methods for osteoporotic bone, probably joint replacement techniques as hemiarthroplasty of the distal humerus or total elbow replacement. Furthermore the treatment of the osteoporosis itself has to be considered in older people [3]. The main goal of the treatment strategy is to restore the complete function of the elbow with free range of motion and free of pain.

Classification

Fractures of the distal humerus can be classified as supracondylar fractures, transcondylar fractures, intercondylar fractures, fractures of the condyles (lateral and medial), fractures of the articular surfaces (capitellum and trochlea), and fractures of the epicondyles.

The most commonly used classification for distal humerus fractures is the AO classification. Three types of fractures are distinguished according to the AO classification.

Type A fractures are extraarticular fractures affecting the apophyse or the metaphyse.

Type B fractures are partiell intraarticular fractures involving just one column (radial or ulnar).

Type C fractures are intraarticular fractures involving the radial and the ulnar column.

A. Berner
Center for Muskuloskeletal Surgery, Charite – University Medicine, Berlin, Germany
e-mail: arne.berner@charite.de

M. L. Nerlich
Department of Trauma Surgery, University Hospital Regensburg, Regensburg, Germany

U. Stöckle
Berufsgenossenschaftliche Unfallklinik Tübingen, Tübingen, Baden-Württemberg, Germany
e-mail: ustoeckle@bgu-tuebingen.de

M. A. E. Gühring (✉)
Klinik im Kronprinzenbau, Reutlingen, Germany
e-mail: dr.guehring@kronprinzenbau-klinik.de

P. Biberthaler et al. (eds.), *Acute Elbow Trauma*, Strategies in Fracture Treatments,
https://doi.org/10.1007/978-3-319-97850-5_3

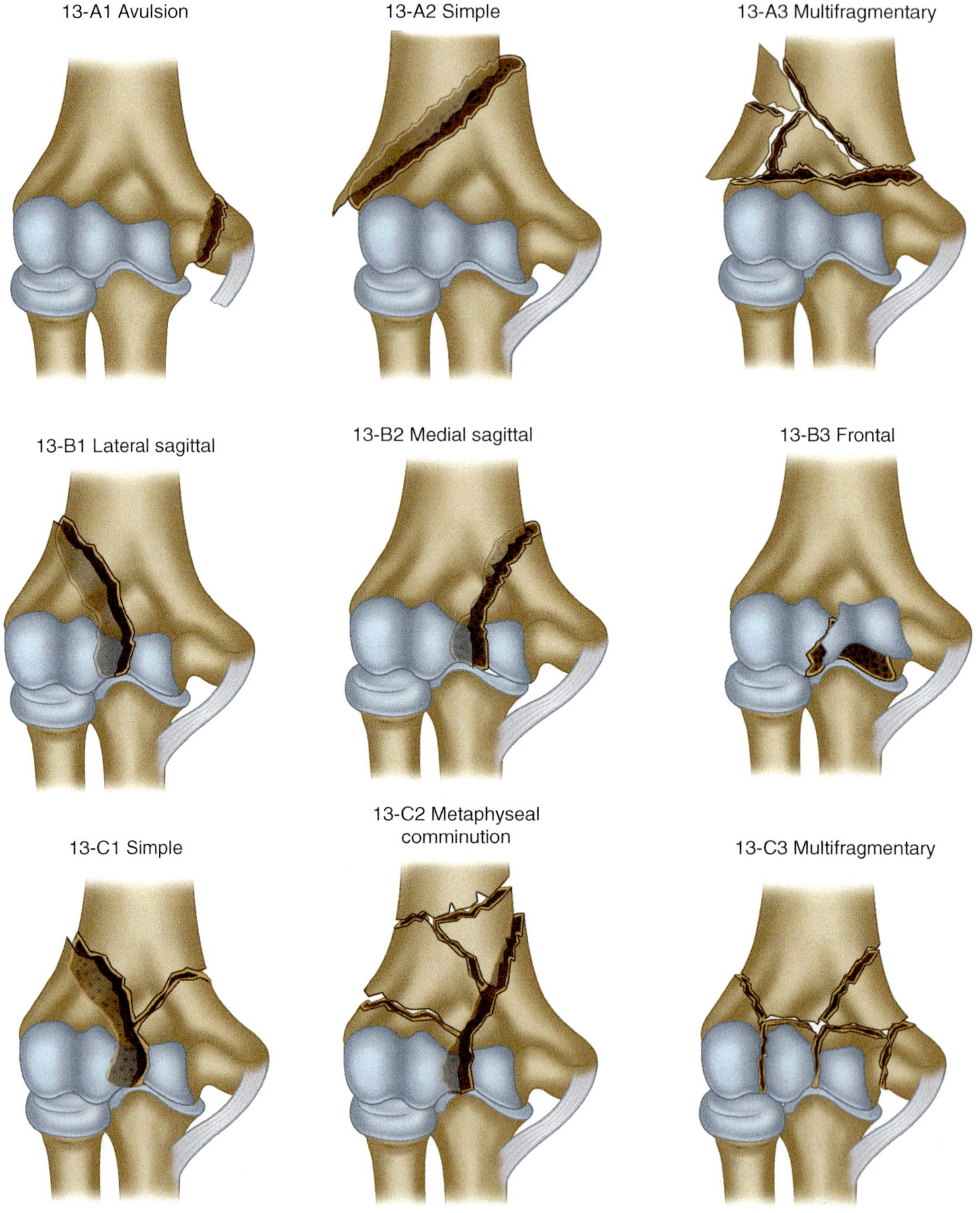

Fig. 3.1 The AO-classification of distal humerus fractures

Table 3.1 Classification of the distal humerus fractures AO type B3 according to Dubberley et al. [4]

Type	Fracture characteristics
I	Fracture of the capitulum with optional inclusion of the lateral border of the trochlea
II	Fracture of the capitulum and the trochlea in one piece
III	Multifragmentary fracture of the trochlea and the capitulum

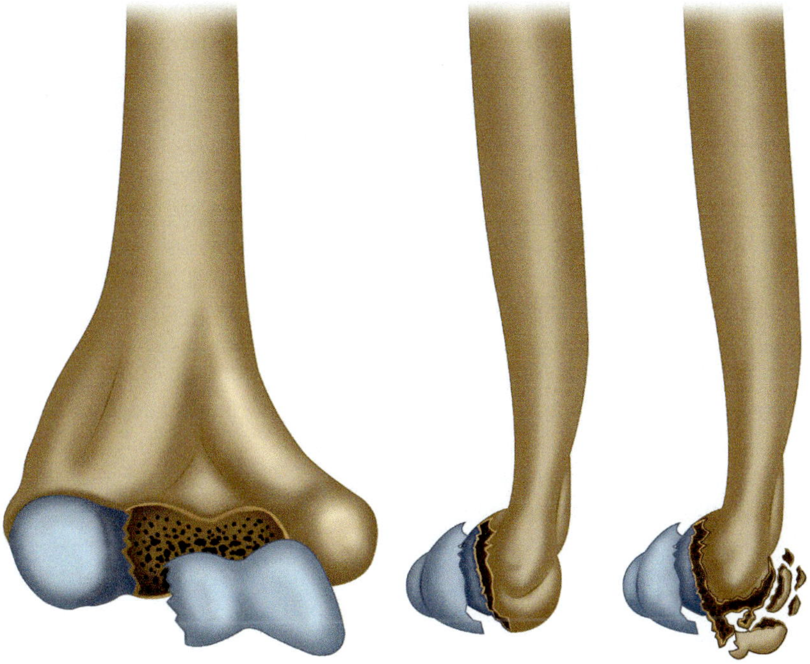

Fig. 3.2 Classification of the distal humerus fractures AO type B3 according to Dubberley et al. [4]

All types are subdivided into three more subtypes (Fig. 3.1).

The type B3 fractures of the distal humerus in the coronal plane are subdivided into three more fracture types of the capitulum and the trochlea according to the dubberley classification (Table 3.1 and Fig. 3.2) [4].

Symptoms and Diagnostics

Patients with distal humeral fractures have severe pain and immobility of the elbow. The contralateral arm is mostly protecting the injured arm. After taking the medical history, the arm is checked for open wounds. The blood supply of the arm is checked and additional vessel and nerve injuries are excluded. Following examination the arm can be protected by a cast and the patient should get adequate pain medication.

The diagnostic procedure starts with an anteroposterior and lateral radiographs. If the fracture pattern still remains unclear on plain radiographs, or in fractures with involvement of the articular surface (type B and C fractures), a computed tomography scan is mandatory to get a better understanding of the fracture and for preoperative planning. In the case of suspected additional vessel injuries, a duplex sonography or a CT angiography has to be performed.

So far, magnetic resonance imaging (MRI) is not very helpful in this kind of fracture diagnostic.

Injury Pattern and Surgery Related Anatomy

Due to the complex anatomy around the elbow and the small soft tissue coverage, we often found open fractures or related injuries of the vessels or nerves. Anatomically, the distal humerus has a triangular shape which contains of two columns [6].

The medial column with the nonarticular medial epicondyle with the insertion of the flexor muscles and the medial part of the humeral trochlea and the lateral column with the capitellum and more proximally the lateral epicondyle with the insertion of the extensor muscles.

From a lateral perspective, the articular surface of the trochlea and capitellum is projected anteriorly at an angle of 40° to the axis of the humerus, the trochlear axis being externally rotated at an angle of 3–8° and compared with the longitudinal axis being in 4–8° of valgus [6, 7].

Non-operative Treatment

Non-operative treatment is very rare because most of the distal humerus fractures are dislocated with anatomical proximity to the joint and need operative treatment.

Non-dislocated fractures can be take into consideration of non-operative approach if a functional treatment of the elbow can be garanteed. However, if the immobilisation period is too long, it may end up in elbow stiffness.

Therefore, non-operative treatment is only indicated in stable and undislocated fractures of the distal humerus, or if the patient has general contraindications for surgery such as severe comorbidities. This widely accepted attitude is supported by the literature which demonstrates high rates of satisfactory outcomes with acceptable complication rates after operative treatment in several studies [8–10].

There are two Level III studies regarding the functional outcomes between operatively and non-operatively treated patients with distal humerus fractures. Nauth et al. performed a pooled analysis of these studies and demonstrated that patients treated non-operatively are almost three times more likely to have an unacceptable result [11, 12]. Another retrospective study by Robinson et al. compared the results in 273 surgically treated patients with those in forty-seven non-operatively treated patients. The authors reported that non-operatively treated patients were almost six times more likely to have a nonunion and four times more likely to have delayed union compared to the operatively treated group [13]. Aitken et al. demonstrated a selection of 40 cases. Short-term results showed 42 points in the Broberg and Morrey score 6 weeks after trauma, and 67 points after 3 months. In long-term follow-ups after 4 years, the mean DASH score in the surviving patients (n = 20) was 38% and 95% had a basic functional flexion of the elbow (mouth to gluteus). Non-union rate 1 year after injury has been reported to be as high as 47% [13].

Therefore, non-operatively treatment of distal humerus fractures is reserved for non-displaced fractures or frail and low-demanding patients. For non-operative treatment, the elbow has to be immobilized in a cast for 2–3 weeks, followed by gentle passive range-of-motion exercises. After 3 weeks, passive exercises start out of the cast. From the sixth week onwards, active elbow motion is allowed. Within these 6 weeks close clinical and neurological monitoring is obligatory and likewise, periodic x-ray controls have to be taken in order to rule out secondary dislocation.

Operative Therapy

Besides the restoration of the joint integrity, the goal of any operative strategy is to enable joint stability and thus functional rehabilitation. The open anatomical joint reduction and internal osteosynthesis according to the principles of the AO represent the current standard care of distal humerus fractures. Percutaneous K-wire osteosynthesis, as well as other minimal procedures, do not achieve primary stability and thus are not adequate care for adults. Whenever possible, the reconstruction of the joint should take place within 24 h after trauma. The early establishment of exercise-stable conditions enables early functional rehabilitation, which is essential for good functional outcomes. Furthermore, this reduces complications such as infection or heterotopic ossification.

Severe soft-tissue injuries, open fractures, vessel or nerve injuries, or a compartment syndrome represent emergency indications that make immediate care indispensable. In an emergency situation, the external fixation of the elbow joint should be preferred.

Surgical Therapy

The selection of the approach depends on the type of planned osteosynthesis. The type of osteosynthesis depends on the morphology of the fracture.

Lateral Approach

The lateral approach is used for:

1. lateral extraarticular fractures (A1.1),
2. partial articular fractures of the lateral epicondyle (B1), and
3. shear fractures of the frontal plane (B3).

The patient is placed in the supine position with an arm table. The skin-incision begins about 3–5 cm proximal of the lateral epicondyle cutting distally along the lower edge of the extensor carpi ulnaris muscle. For further dissection, one must look out for the cutaneus antebrachii posterior nerve. It runs epifascially ca. 2 cm ventral of the lateral epicondyle in a distal direction. Subcutaneous tissue is split. After identification of the fascia, it will be opened between the extensor carpi ulnaris and the anconeus muscle. Immediately appears the joint capsule, which is then split along its length. The lateral access can be extended proximally by identifying and splitting the lateral intermusculare septum and disecting away the brachioradialis muscle and also the extensor carpi radialis longus muscle subperiostal toward the bending side.

Medial Approach

The medial approach is used for:

1. ulnar-side, extraarticular fractures (A1.2) and
2. partial articular fractures of the medial epicondyle (B2).

The patient is placed in the supine position with an arm table. The skin-incision runs from ca. 5 cm proximal to ca. 10 cm distal of the medial epicondyle. After splitting the subcutaneous tissue, the medial intermusculare septum will be sought out. It spans from the medial epicondyle along the supracondylar crest proximally and divides the extension from the flexion muscle mass. In this area, one must pay attention to the medial cutaneus antebrachial nerve, which runs epifascially. In the further dissection, the ulnar nerve should be presented proximally and followed in a distal direction up to the departure of the first motor branch. The muscle group is now split along the medial intermuscular septum until the joint capsule appears. The joint capsule is then also split along its length.

Dorsal Approaches

The dorsal approach represents the standard approach, since the entire joint can be exposed from the dorsal side. Both the medial and also the lateral approach can be reached from dorsally. So the dorsal approach must be seen as the one from which the deep approach can be carried out without supplemental skin-incisions. A further advantage of the dorsal approach is that the critical neurovascular structures, which are placed on the bending side, cannot be endangered, except the ulnar nerve on the medial side. The central point for the dorsal approach is the question of how the triceps brachii muscle will be handled. Altogether, four basic principles can be differentiated, in which the muscle is either split centrally ("Triceps Splitting"), pushed to the side ("Triceps Reflecting") or removed by osteotomy of the olecranon. The fourth operation technique maintains the triceps attachment points with medial and lateral dissection past the muscle in the direction of the joint (paratricipital approach). For the dorsal approach, the patient can be placed either prone with removal of the affected arm or in a lateral position. In the lateral position, the arm is placed on the chest and held by a second assistant on the opposite side. For operative procedure an elbow flexion of more than 90° is mandatory.

The skin-incision starts proximally to the tip of the olecranon and proceeds distally. The olecranon should be circumscribed on the radial side, in order to avoid wound healing complications. In the region of the olecranon, the skin-incision should be applied up to the fascia. In this way, the blood supply of the medial and lateral soft-tissue flaps should be optimized and thus the risk of wound healing disorders reduced. After the fascia is dissected, the ulnar nerve must be identified proximally and, depending on the indication, followed distally until the first motor branch.

Olecranon Osteotomy

After soft-tissue dissection, a chevron-form incision of the bone is carried out in the area of the olecranon with an oscillating saw, whereby the chevron is open in the proximal direction. The completion of the osteotomy is carried out with the chisel, in order to produce negligible loss of bone from the olecranon, so repositioning of the olecranon during withdrawal is made easier. Furthermore, it is recommendable to end the osteotomy in the histological bare-zone of the olecranon, in order to not unnecessarily destroy joint cartilage. The vertex of the planned chevron can be marked with a Kirschner wire or a drill bit as desired. The osteotomy takes place from the vertex of the chevron outward in an angle of 40°. After cutting through the olecranon, the extension structures and the distal humerus are dissected and removed proximally. This enables a good view to the joint. An extension of the approach is possible by removal of the collateral ligaments. During dissection of the triceps proximally, one must pay attention to the crossing radial nerve. After completing the reconstruction of the joint surfaces, an exercise-stable osteosynthesis must be carried out in the area of the olecranonosteotomy. Various possibilities for the osteosynthesis are available to the surgeon. Regardless of the form of osteosynthesis (tension band wiring, angle-stable plate osteosynthesis, or intramedular screws), a step-free reposition of the osteotomy cleft has to be restored.

Triceps Splitting Approach

The incision for splitting the triceps begins ca. 8 cm proximal to the tip of the olecranon and then runs centrally over the tip on the edge of the ulna for about 4–5 cm in the distal direction. The triceps tendon passes medial into the flexor fascia and lateral into the fascia of the anconeus and the extensor muscles. This anatomical region must be preserved through sharp subperiosteal dissection on the bones. Both parts of the triceps are mobilized now until, depending on the indication, an exarticulation of the joint is possible. Alternatively, a thin bone flake underneath the tendon can also be removed in the area of the olecranon. After the osteosynthesis a secure attachment of the detached triceps tendon is essential. Transosseous stitches are recommended for this. They can, for example, be tightly attached to the dorsal edge of the ulna with a 2.0 mm drill.

Triceps Reflecting Approach According to Bryan and Morrey

After identification and release of the ulnar nerve, the triceps insertion is detached from the proximal ulna subperiosteally with the entire lower arm fascia from medial to lateral. The anconeus muscle is detached subperiosteally on the lateral edge of the ulna, and thus is raised in continuity with the extension structures. After cutting through the medial collateral ligament, the joint can be dislodged. If applicable, a release of the lateral collateral ligament is also necessary for that. As in the triceps splitting access, a bony sliver in the area of the olecranon can also be detached here. During withdrawal, the ligaments must be securely attached. Likewise, the reconstruction of the extension structures onto the olecranon must be given attention and transosseous stitches must be applied.

Paratricipital Approach

Both, the medial and the lateral intermuscular septum are sought out and the ulnar nerve is secured. Proximally, the ulnar nerve is followed along its course on the medial intermuscular septum, and the triceps muscle is mobilized radially. The triceps fascia is split, and the muscle is mobilized from the lateral intermuscular septum and humerus towards the ulnar side. The entire triceps muscle is isolated using a gauze wrap. This permits the whole triceps muscle to be moved towards either the lateral or medial side, in order to get access to the distal humerus.

At the level of the joint, the collateral ligaments and the origins of the extensors and flexors can be detached, if this facilitates the procedure. The triceps-on approach provides only a limited representation of the joint. After osteosynthesis the refixation of the lateral ligaments and the muscle groups is mandatory.

Osteosynthesis Procedures

External Fixation

Besides extensive open or closed soft-tissue damage, the main indications for the use of external fixation are residual instability or polytraumatized patients. The function of the external fixation is to establish quickly and temporarily a stable position of the elbow joint. The application takes place most often in the supine position. External fixation is only of limited suitability for the treatment of distal humerus fractures, since an anatomical reduction is not possible and because a long position of rest is accompanied by substantial limitations of movement in the region of the elbow joint. Therefore, the function of external fixation is temporary stabilization until the prerequisites exist for internal osteosynthesis. The standard construct consists the placing of two Schanz screws in the humerus and the ulna. In the region of the humerus shaft, attention must be paid to the radial nerve. The Schanz screws are inserted proximal to the crossing of the radial nerve anterolateraly. Sufficiently large skin-incisions with blunt dissection of the bones and insertion of drilling sleeves are indispensable for the protection of the nerves.

With the forearm in neutral position, Schanz screws are inserted from a posterolateral aspect directly to the proximal third of the ulna. It is an easily recognizable and palpable bone. The radius shaft should only be included for limitation of the rotation movement of the forearm. If the fixation is installed in the three tube modular technique it can easily switch to movement fixation, in cases of persisting instability, by installing a movement bracket.

K-wire Osteosynthesis

Osteosynthesis of fractures of the distal humerus by means of Kirschner wires remain reserved essentially for pediatric fractures.

Screw Osteosynthesis

Isolated screw osteosynthesis without support from a plate is only indicated for partial intraarticular fractures or avulsion injuries of the epidcondyles. Screw osteosynthesis of the small fragment instruments with canulated screw systems are available in different sizes. According to the rules of osteosynthesis, it is recommended to use two screws, which are inserted in parallel or diverging, in order to ensure rotational stability. When treating complex multi-fragment fractures or especially shear fractures in the frontal plane, head-sinking mini-screws (2.0 mm) are used, so the head of the screw lies deep to the surface of the joint cartilage.

Nail Osteosynthesis

Nail osteosynthesis can be used for treatment of type A2 and type 3 fractures, if the distal fragment is large enough. The advantage of nail osteosynthesis is generally the minimally invasive application. The disadvantage of the anterograde nail osteosynthesis is the compromising of the rotator cuffs. In cases of short distal fracture fragments, a rotation-stable fixation of the nail with two locking bolts is especially difficult. Therefore, nail osteosynthesis is not the first choice of therapy for treatment of distal humerus fractures.

Plate Osteosynthesis

Angular stable plating is established as the gold standard for the treatment of distal intraarticular humerus fractures. Helfet and Hotchkiss were able to show a significant higher stabilitiy with double plating, in comparison to screw osteosynthesis or single plates, regardless of the type of plate (1/3 tube-plate or reconstruction plate) [14].

In recent years, new plate fixation systems (LCP®, Synthes) have been developed specially for this fracture entity. Anatomically precontoured and angular stable plates offer new perspectives in fracture care in cases of metaphyseal shatter/defect situations, complex joint destruction and osteoporosis. These plates are also available as polyaxial systems. The plates are configured with conventional or angle-stable 3.5 mm screws in the proximal area and 2.7 mm screws in the distal area. The dorsolateral plate also offers the possibility of inserting screws in lateromedial direction through the lateral epicondyle to stabilize the articular mass. Due to the anatomical preformation, shorter operating times can be achieved, which justifies the higher costs of the implant. While a one-sided plate osteosynthesis is sufficient in cases of partial articular fractures (B1 and B2) and metaphyseal fractures (A2 and A3). Intraarticular fractures (C1–3) have to be stabilized through a double-plate construct. Above all, the correct positioning of the two plates to each other – whether in so-called 90° or 180° orientation – is currently debated. The parallel arrangement shows a significant advantage when using non-angle-stable plate systems [15]. In comparisons of the angle-stable implants though, no significant difference between these two arrangements has been found so far [16]. The disadvantage of the parallel arrangement is the both-sided application of the implants and possible blocking of the screws crossing each other. In the application of both plates, the dorsolateral (radial) plate should be selected two screw-holes longer in the proximal direction, in order to avoid stress concentration.

Fracture-Specific Care

A functional restoration of the elbow joint is only possible if through an anatomical joint reconstruction a stable fracture and ligament situation is restored. Correspondingly, awareness of the fracture classification is of decisive importance for the preoperative planning, since the osteosynthesis procedure is dependent on the type of fracture.

Supracondylar Fractures (AO Classification AO 13-A2 and AO 13-A3)

The standard care of metaphyseal fractures on the distal humerus is double plating osteosynthesis. For supracondylar distal humerus fractures, the paratricipital approach should be chosen, in which the extension apparatus is preserved. Anatomically preformed, angle-stable locking plates are applied, which are fitted in 90° technique (radial-dorsal and ulnar-lateral) or in parallel technique depending on surgeons preference (Fig. 3.3). At least two screws for each plate should be applied in the proximal and distal main fragments to assure sufficient primary stability.

Epicondylar Fractures (AO Classification AO 13-A1)

Fractures of the lateral and medial epicondyle are avulsion injuries with bony tearing out of the ligaments. Corresponding to the muscle pull dislocation of the fragment can be expected, so that even slightly displaced fragments should be fixed. The fragments can be repositioned via lateral or medial approach and refixed by means of screw osteosynthesis. If the size of the fragments allows, at least two screws or one screw and one K-wire should be applied in order to increase the rotational stability of the fragment (Fig. 3.4). For avulsion fractures in the area of the medial epicondyle the course of the ulnar nerve must be heeded.

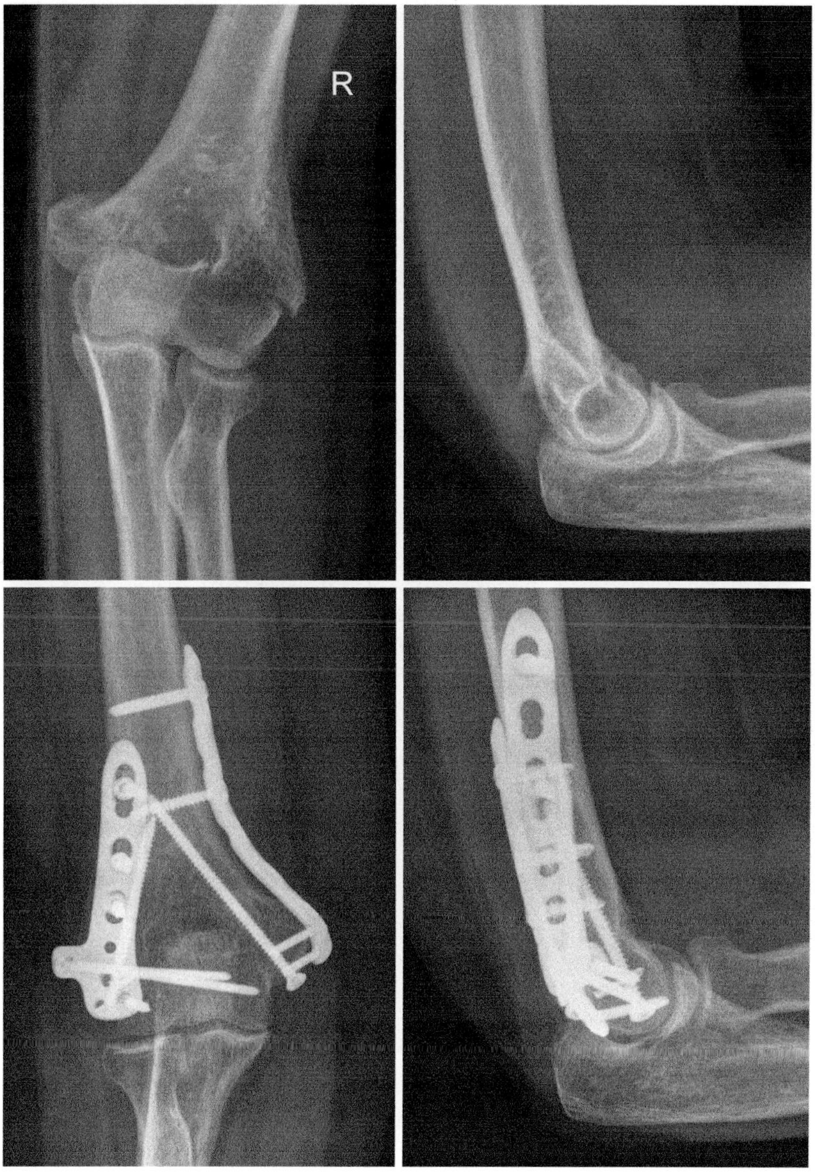

Fig. 3.3 Supracondyle fracture (AO 13-A2). Traditional 90-90 plating technique with column screws. Paratricipital approach

Partial Articular Unicondylar Fractures (AO Classification AO 13-B1 and 13-B2)

Depending on their position, fractures can be treated via a lateral or medial approach. A stable osteosynthesis can be achieved through primary screw osteosynthesis with interfragmentary compression in combination with an angle-stable plate osteosynthesis as neutralization plates. Especially for osteoporotic bones, the application of a single screw osteosynthesis is obsolete, because of the poor bone quality and resulting elevated rate of secondary dislocation.

Partial Articular Frontal Fractures/ Shear Fracturen (AO 13-B3)

To visualize the entirety of this complex fracture type the additional medial approach is necessary quite often besides the "standard"

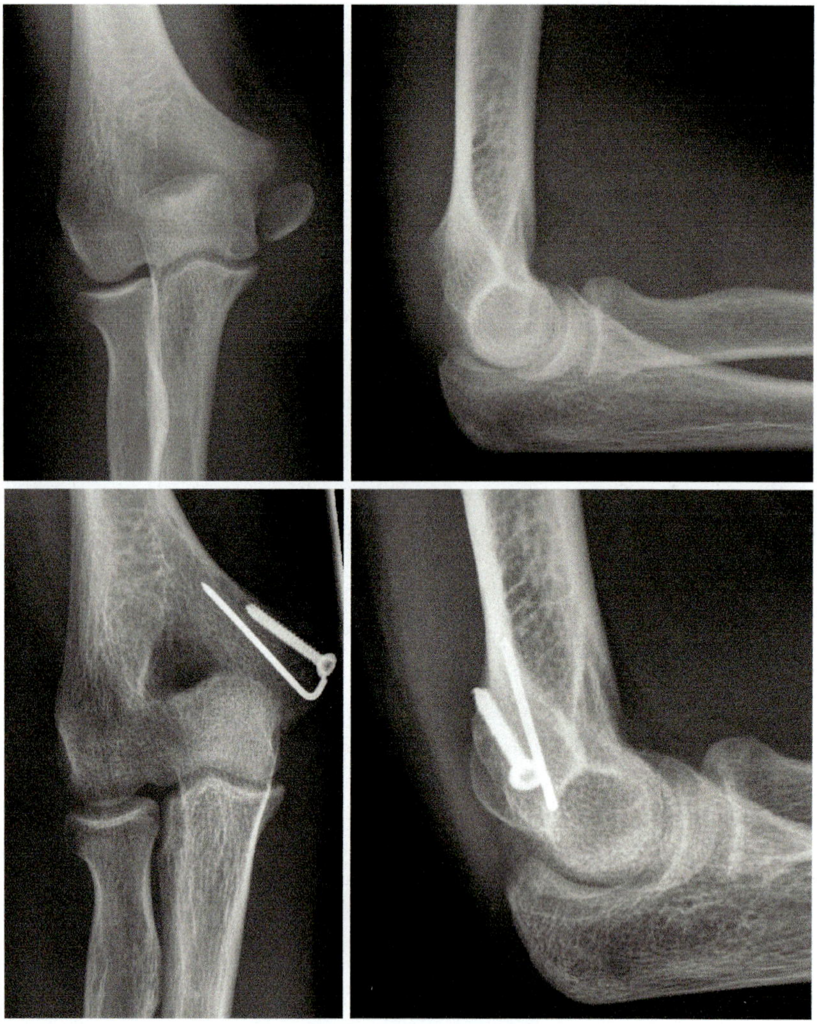

Fig. 3.4 Fracture of the radial epicondyle (AO 13-A1). Open reduction and fixation with small fragment screw and K-wire

lateral approach. For these fractures a CT-scan with 3D-reconstruction is essential for preoperative planning to understand the fracture severity. After anatomic repositioning of the fracture, the reduction can be fixated preliminarily by means of Kirschner wires and then, depending on the fracture morphology, the osteosynthesis can be stabilized osteosynthetically from the joint side by means of countersunk mini-screws (2.0 mm) (Fig. 3.5). Depending on the size of the capitulum fragments, the reduction can be secured from the extension side by using dorsoradial plates with anteriorly directed screws.

Complete Articular Fractures

The goal of the osteosynthesis for intraarticular fractures is the step-free restoration of the humeral joint surface. Regardless of the approach, angle-stable plating systems have established themselves. In the classic procedure, the articular surface should first be repositioned and fixed. The intact ulna and radius can be used as a template for the correct length and orientation. The joint-carrying fragments are preliminarily held by means of K-wires in order to be treated with a compression osteosynthesis. Here there is the possibility of per-

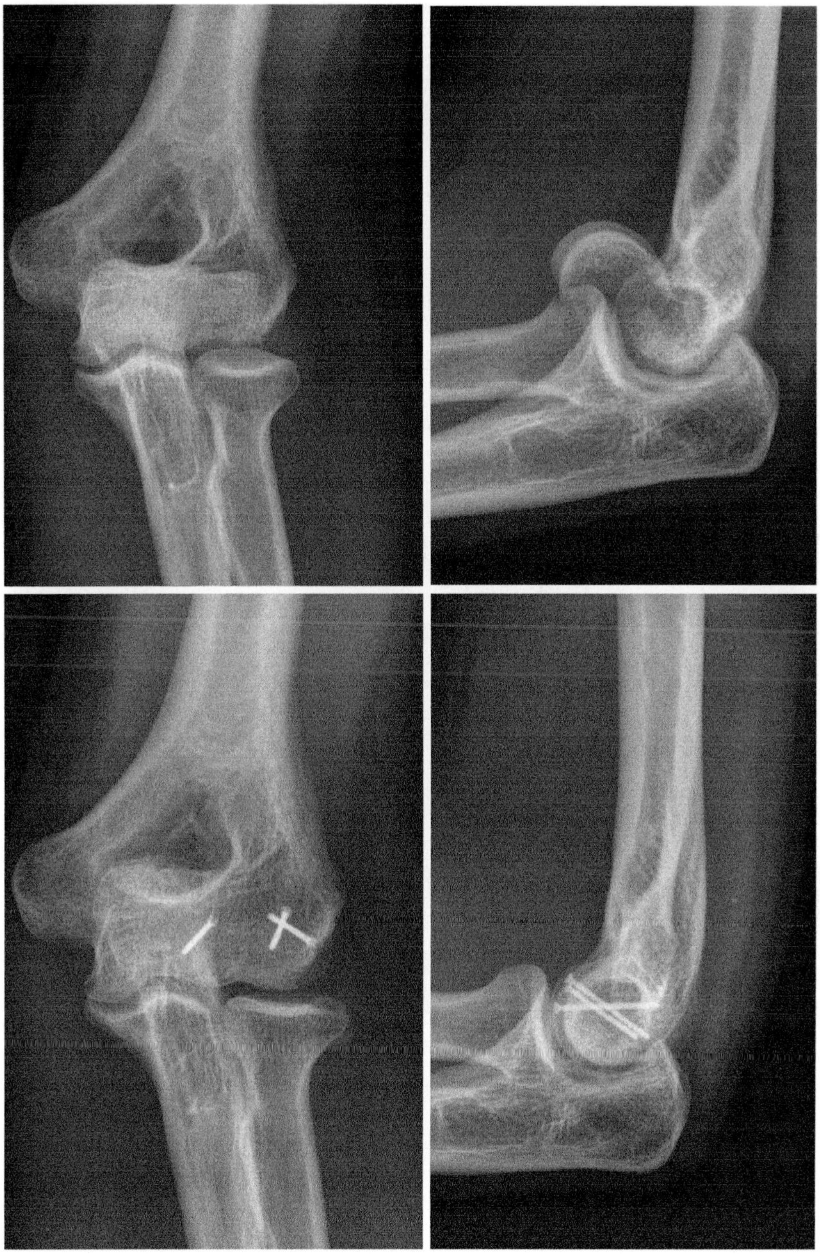

Fig. 3.5 Shear fracture of the distal humerus (AO 13-B3). Open reduction and fixation with countersunk mini-screws

forming an interfragmentary tension screw osteosynthesis from the radial side. The screws should run parallel to the joint line. After stabilization of the articular mass, it can now be fixed by column screws and/or angle-stable plate systems against the shaft (Fig. 3.6). Depending on the fracture morphology and a possible bony defect situation in the metaphyseal portion, a shortening osteosynthesis can be accepted here (Fig. 3.7). Alternately, in

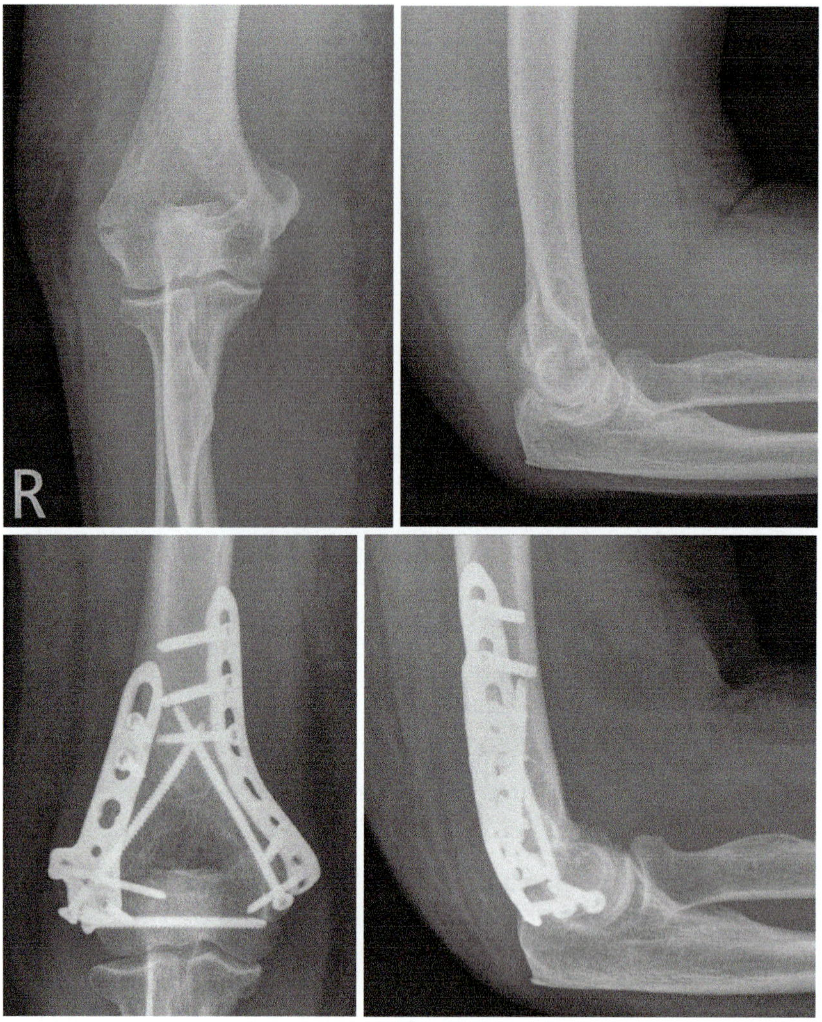

Fig. 3.6 Supraintercondyle fracture (AO 13-C1). Traditional 90-90 plating technique with column screws after fixation of the articular mass with screw running parallel to the joint line. Paratricipital approach

cases of pronounced metaphyseal defect zones, an autologous bone grafting (harvested from the dorsal iliac crest) can be performed. The length of the plates should allow for at least three bicortical screws into the proximal main fragment (shaft) (Fig. 3.8). Furthermore, a stress concentration on the proximal end of the plates should be avoided through the use of identical plate lengths.

Care of Elderly Patients

Even for geriatric patients the anatomical reconstruction of the joint with sufficient stability has to be the primary therapeutic goal, thus providing the prerequisite for early functional rehabilitation and especially for daily activities (handling the walker). Primary stability in osteoporotic bones can be achieved through the use of angular stable

Fig. 3.7 Complex distal humerus fracture with open soft-tissue damage (AO 13-C2). Open reduction and shortening osteosynthesis because of the defect situation in the metaphyseal portion

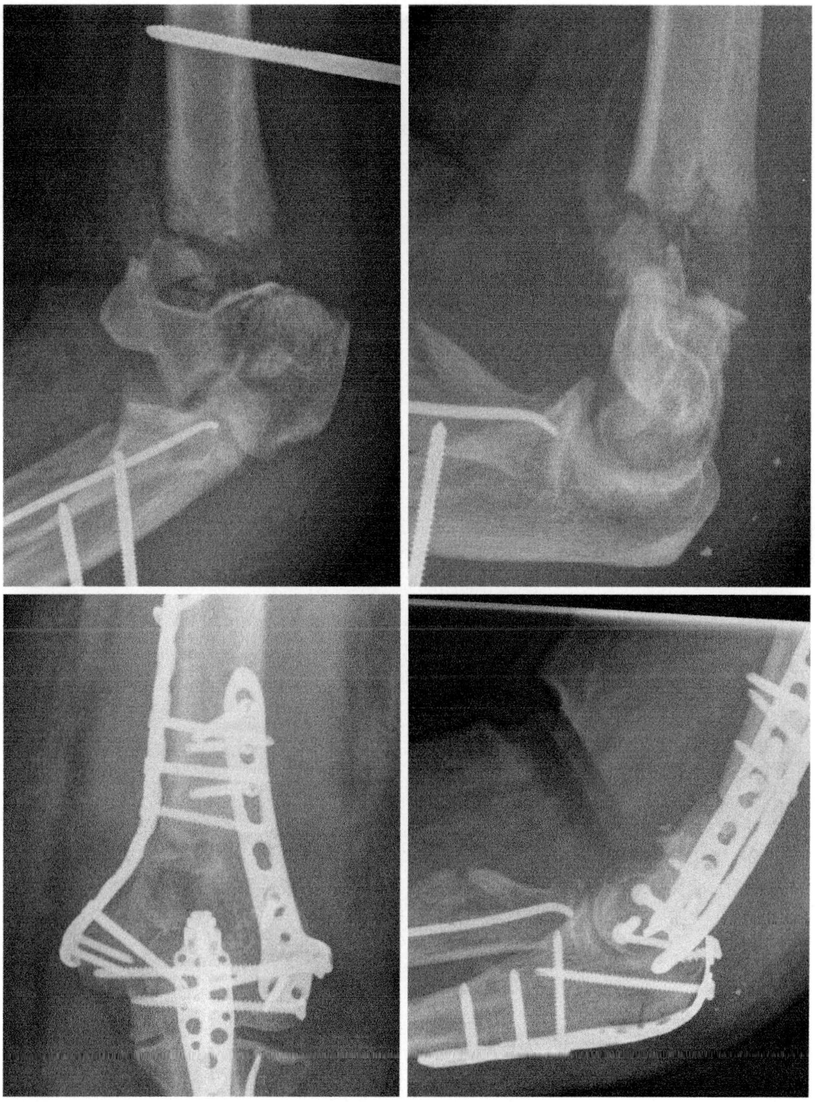

osteosynthesis [17, 18]. Most complications are the loss of thereduction with implant failure due to poor bone quality. Therefore in exceptional cases a postoperative immobilization, a corresponding orthesis or a supplemental installation of a movement fixator is possible. If reconstruction is not possible due to the complexity of the fracture or the bone quality, then the joint replacement is indicated.

Rehabilitation

For the earliest mobilization of the elbow joint, in order to avoid stiffness the physiotherapy regime conforms accordingly to the intraoperatively achieved stability. After immobilization of the elbow joint in the operating room by means of an upper arm splint or an elbow orthesis, the first replacing of the cast and the x-ray control are

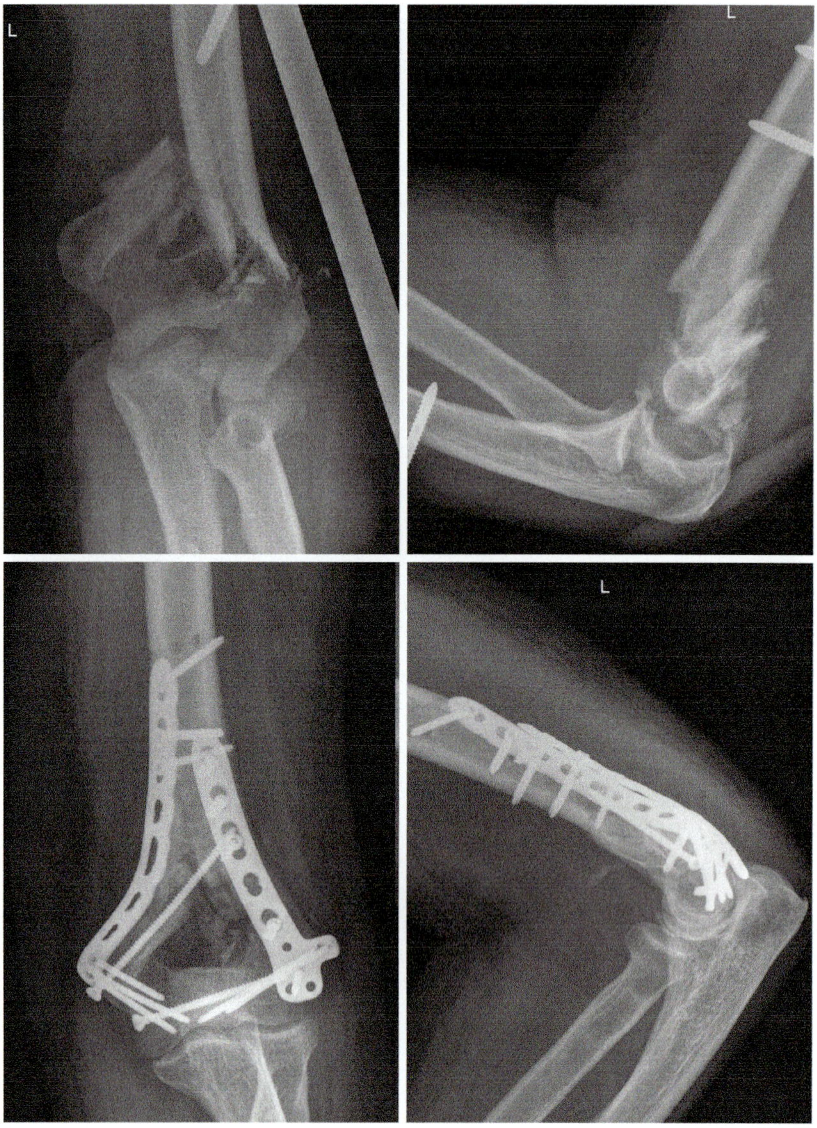

Fig. 3.8 Complex distal humerus fracture (AO 13-C3). Traditional 90-90 plating technique. Paratricipital approach

carried out on the second post-operative day. In correct progress, active and passive movement can take place under physiotherapeutic surveillance already from the second postoperative day onward. The orthesis or the upper arm cast can be, depending on the specifications of the surgeon, increasingly omitted during the day, but it should be worn at night for 6 weeks postoperatively. Strain of the elbow in regards to lifting and carrying, as well as axial supporting, should be avoided for a total of 6 weeks postoperatively. Beside an adequate pain therapy, cryotherapy can reduce the subjective pain sensitivity. Measures to reduce swelling take place by an AV-pump, as well as elevated resting and lymph drainage. A possible later limitation of joint movement be caused by formation of heterotopic ossification. Accordingly, ossification prophylaxis is routinely carried out by means of Indometacin 50 1–0–1 for 14 days.

Postoperative Complications

Complications in the treatment of distal humerus fractures occur at rates of up to 30% [19]. Differentiations must be made between:

Heterotopic Ossification

Clinically relevant heterotopic ossification resulting in restriction of elbow ROM is described in the literature for 14% of the cases [20]. For prevention of heterotopic ossification, ossification prophylaxis by means of Indometacin 50 mg 2/d should take place already on the day of the accident for the period of 14 days.

Nerve Damage

While the radial nerve represents the most frequently affected nerve for primary traumatic lesions, iatrogenic injury of the ulnar nerve is the most dreaded intraoperative and postoperative complication [19]. In order to avoid an intraoperative lesion of the ulnar nerve, it has proven worthwhile to protect that nerve at the beginning of the operation during the soft tissue dissection and to follow it distally until the first motor branch. If no mechanical irritation of the nerve is expected from the osteosynthesis or bones, the nerve can remain in its original position. Otherwise the nerve should be transpositioned to anterior in a subcutaneous layer by resecting the intermuscular septum.

Elbow Stiffness

The functional arc according to Morrey describes a range of motion for extension/flexion of 0–30–130° and for pronation/supination of 50–0–50° as the range of motion with which 90% of the activities of everyday life can be carried out [21]. Among the causes of elbow stiffness, a differentiation is made between factors that are extrinsic (heterotopic ossification, capsular fibrosis, muscular contractions) versus intrinsic (osteophytes, joint congruence, adhesions). Mostly there are mixed causes. Early functional rehabilitation is necessary to avoid elbow stiffness. The prerequisite for early functional rehabilitation is a stable osteosynthesis. Before any operative arthrolysis is indicated (arthroscopic or open) every possible nonoperative therapy measure should be exhausted and the cause of the restricted motion should be evaluated precisely.

Infections

The rate of infection depends on the initial soft tissue trauma and the timing of care. Postoperative infections are reported in the literature in 12% of the cases after surgical treatment of a distal humerus fracture [22]. Clinical signs of infection are disrupted wound healing, redness, swelling, and putrid discharge. If an infection is present, priority is given to decontamination of the infection with removal of any implanted osteosynthesis material, as well as transfixation of the elbow joint, if needed, by means of external fixation.

Pseudoarthrosis

Delayed or non-union is a rare complication for distal humerus fractures and is described in the literature with an incidence of 2–10% [23]. The goal of revision surgery has to be functional reconstruction of the joint, which can be achieved through a reosteosynthesis combined with additional bone graft. For elderly patients with poor bone quality and possible secondary dislocation of the primary osteosynthesis, arthroplasty should be considered as an alternative.

References

1. Robinson CM, Hill RM, Jacobs N, Dall G, Court-Brown CM. Adult distal humeral metaphyseal fractures: epidemiology and results of treatment. J Orthop Trauma. 2003;17:38–47.

2. Palvanen M, Kannus P, Niemi S, Parkkari J. Secular trends in distal humeral fractures of elderly women: nationwide statistics in Finland between 1970 and 2007. Bone. 2010;46:1355–8.
3. Nauth A, McKee MD, Ristevski B, Hall J, Schemitsch EH. Distal humeral fractures in adults. J Bone Joint Surg Am. 2011;93:686–700.
4. Dubberley JH, Faber KJ, Macdermid JC, Patterson SD, King GJ. Outcome after open reduction and internal fixation of capitellar and trochlear fractures. J Bone Joint Surg Am. 2006;88:46–54.
5. Goncalves LB, Ring DC. Fractures of the humeral trochlea: case presentations and review. J Shoulder Elb Surg. 2016;25:e151–5.
6. Jupiter JB, Mehne DK. Fractures of the distal humerus. Orthopedics. 1992;15:825–33.
7. Anglen J. Distal humerus fractures. J Am Acad Orthop Surg. 2005;13:291–7.
8. Atalar AC, Demirhan M, Salduz A, Kilicoglu O, Seyahi A. Functional results of the parallel-plate technique for complex distal humerus fractures. Acta Orthop Traumatol Turc. 2009;43:21–7.
9. Theivendran K, Duggan PJ, Deshmukh SC. Surgical treatment of complex distal humeral fractures: functional outcome after internal fixation using precontoured anatomic plates. J Shoulder Elb Surg. 2010;19:524–32.
10. Sanchez-Sotelo J, Torchia ME, O'Driscoll SW. Complex distal humeral fractures: internal fixation with a principle-based parallel-plate technique. J Bone Joint Surg Am. 2007;89:961–9.
11. Srinivasan K, Agarwal M, Matthews SJ, Giannoudis PV. Fractures of the distal humerus in the elderly: is internal fixation the treatment of choice? Clin Orthop Relat Res. 2005;434:222–30.
12. Zagorski JB, Jennings JJ, Burkhalter WE, Uribe JW. Comminuted intraarticular fractures of the distal humeral condyles. Surgical vs. nonsurgical treatment. Clin Orthop Relat Res. 1986;202:197–204.
13. Aitken SA, Jenkins PJ, Rymaszewski L. Revisiting the 'bag of bones': functional outcome after the conservative management of a fracture of the distal humerus. Bone Joint J. 2015;97-B:1132–8.
14. Helfet DL, Hotchkiss RN. Internal fixation of the distal humerus: a biomechanical comparison of methods. J Orthop Trauma. 1990;4:260–4.
15. Arnander MW, Reeves A, MacLeod IA, et al. A biomechanical comparison of plate configuration in distal humerus fractures. J Orthop Trauma. 2008;22:332–6.
16. Shin SJ, Sohn HS, Do NH. A clinical comparison of two different double plating methods for intraarticular distal humerus fractures. J Shoulder Elbow Surg. 2010;19:2–9.
17. Korner J, Diederichs G, Arzdorf M, et al. A biomechanical evaluation of methods of distal humerus fracture fixation using locking compression plates versus conventional reconstruction plates. J Orthop Trauma. 2004;18:286–93.
18. Voigt C, Rank C, Waizner K, et al. Biomechanical testing of a new plate system for the distal humerus compared to two well-established implants. Int Orthop. 2013;37:667–72.
19. Jupiter JB. Complex fractures of the distal part of the humerus and associated complications. Instr Course Lect. 1995;44:187–98.
20. Douglas K, Cannada LK, Archer KR, et al. Incidence and risk factors of heterotopic ossification following major elbow trauma. Orthopedics. 2012;35:e815–22.
21. Clement H, Pichler W, Tesch NP, et al. Anatomical basis of the risk of radial nerve injury related to the technique of external fixation applied to the distal humerus. Surg Radiol Anat. 2010;32:221–4.
22. Chen NC, Julka A. Hinged external fixation of the elbow. Hand Clin. 2010;26:423–33, vii.
23. Siebenlist S, Reeps C, Kraus T, et al. Brachial artery transection caused by closed elbow dislocation in a mature in-line skater: a case report with review of the literature. Knee Surg Sports Traumatol Arthrosc. 2010;18:1667–70.

Proximal Ulna Fractures

4

Kilian Wegmann, Michael Hackl, and Klaus J. Burkhart

Epidemiology

The exposed subcutaneous location makes the olecranon prone to fractures. Olecranon fractures pose a disruption of the extensor mechanism (Fig. 4.1) with potentially severe restriction of elbow function – e.g. reaching over the head or push off from a chair etc. Olecranon fractures are common adult fractures and account for approximately 10–20% of all elbow fractures [1, 2]. Simple displaced fractures represent the most common fracture type. The incidence was estimated as 1.08 per 10.000 person-years [1]. A direct impact due to a fall on the flexed elbow poses the most common fracture mechanism [3]. On the other hand, indirect forces may lead to an olecranon fracture due to the pull of the triceps. There is no predominance of male or female gender but men suffer proximal ulna fractures at a younger age and often present with more complex fracture pattern due to a high energy trauma. Especially in older female patients olecranon fractures may result from a low energy trauma complicated by poor bone quality.

Classification

The Mayo classification [4] (Fig. 4.2) is simple and reproducible. Furthermore, treatment recommendations can be derived from the different fracture types. Therefore, the Mayo classification is the most commonly used in clinical practice. Three different fracture types are described:

Type I:	undisplaced fractures	5%
Type II:	displaced fractures with a stable elbow	85%
Type III:	displaced fractures associated with elbow instability	10%
(e.g. transolecranon dislocation fractures, Monteggia- and Monteggia-like lesions)		

Each fracture type is further devided into simple (A) and comminuted (B) fracture types. According to Colton et al. fractures with a displacement less than 2 mm are considered type I fractures [5]. Type I A and B fractures can be considered the same entity as there is no significant displacement.

The AO classification [6] (Fig. 4.3) is difficult and does not give treatment recommendations. Its clinical use is therefore inapplicable.

K. Wegmann (✉) · M. Hackl
Department of Orthopedic and Trauma Surgery, University Hospital of Cologne, Cologne, Germany
e-mail: Kilian.Wegmann@uk-koeln.de; Michael.hackl@uk-koeln.de

K. J. Burkhart
Arcus Sportklinik, Pforzheim, Germany

P. Biberthaler et al. (eds.), *Acute Elbow Trauma*, Strategies in Fracture Treatments,
https://doi.org/10.1007/978-3-319-97850-5_4

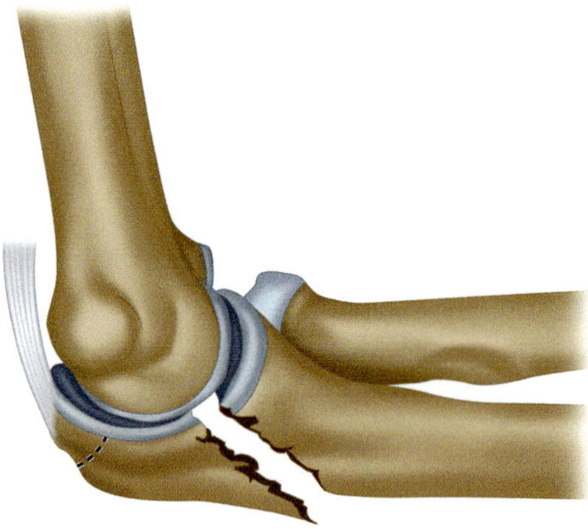

Fig. 4.1 Olecranonfractures pose a disruption of the extensor mechanism

Symptoms and Diagnostics

Clinical examination of a patient with a suspected proximal ulna fracture starts with careful inspection in order to rule out any open wounds. Due to the thin soft tissue coverage of the olecranon these fractures often present as open fractures. The fracture may be visible at first sight in skinny patients. If not, gentle palpation may be performed searching for a fracture gap and potential concomitant injuries such as a radial head fracture. If the fracture is not identified on first sight, integrity of the extensor mechanism is tested by asking the patient to extend the elbow over the head. Any neurovascular injury has to be excluded; especially the ulnar nerve has to be

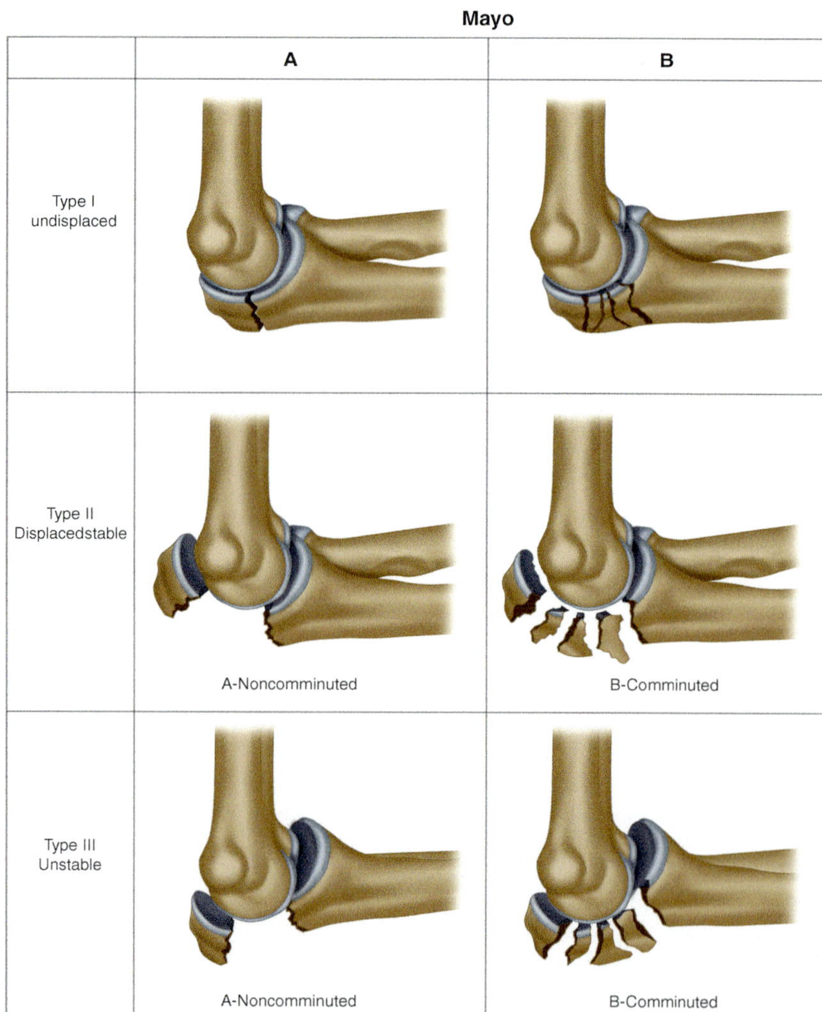

Fig. 4.2 Mayo classification of olecranon fractures

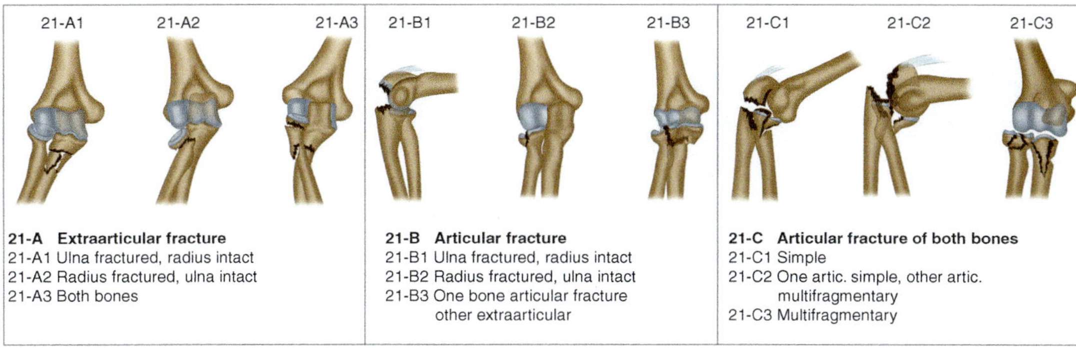

Fig. 4.3 AO-classification of proximal forarm fractures

checked because of its proximity to the proximal ulna.

Plain a.p. and lateral radiographs are sufficient in simple olecranon fractures. However, concomitant radial head, sublime tubercle and coronoid fractures have to be excluded. In case of more complex fractures a CT scan with 2D and 3D reconstructions are mandatory. The CT scan has useful proven in recognizing an intermediate articular fragment.

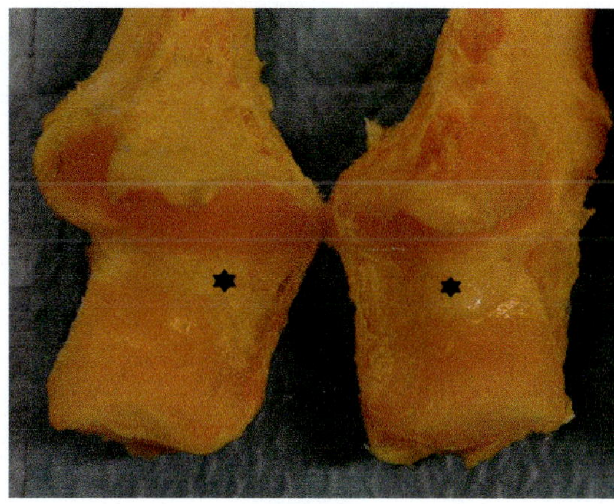

Fig. 4.4 The figure displays the bare area (lighter areas, marked with stars) in two different specimens. Note the variability of the shape and size of the bare area

Injury Pattern and Surgery Related Anatomy

Simple olecranon fractures (Mayo I & II) involve the semilunar or greater sigmoid notch, which is formed by the coronoid process and olecranon. These are separated by the "bare area", which is devoid of cartilage (Fig. 4.4). Reconstructing an olecranon fracture, the bare area must be strictly respected otherwise the greater sigmoid notch will be narrowed resulting in a mismatch with the trochlea (Fig. 4.5).

More complex fracture patterns of the proximal ulna (Mayo III) comprise transolecranon fracture dislocations and monteggia fractures and monteggia like lesions:

- Transolecranon fracture dislocation: proximal ulna fracture with anterior dislocation of the ulnohumeral joint, but intact proximal radioulnar joint (PRUJ).
- Monteggia fracture: proximal ulna fracture with dislocation of the PRUJ, but without ulnohumeral dislocation (cross reference to Monteggia fractures)
- Monteggia like lesion: Monteggia fracture with additional fracture of the dislocated radial head. (cross reference to Monteggia fractures)

Besides the olecranon, transolecranon fracture dislocations often comprise key structures of elbow stability such as the coronoid process, sublime tubercle and supinator crest:

- The olecranon prevents anterior dislocation of the forearm. Furthermore it is an important stabiliser against varus and valgus forces – especially in the

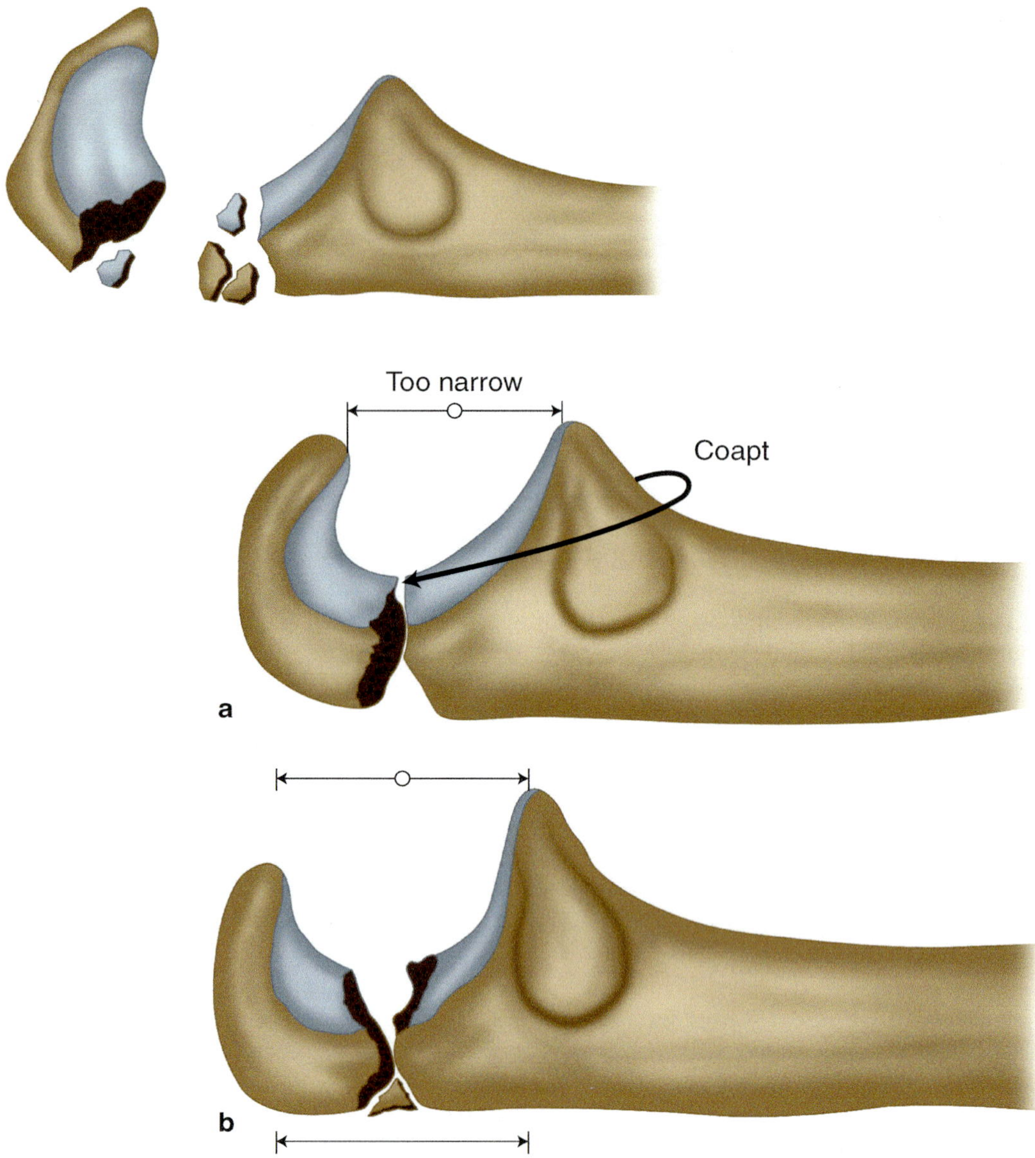

Fig. 4.5 Importance of correct alignement of olecranon farcture reduction

extended elbow. The triceps insertion omits the olecranon tip allowing the tip to dive into the fossa in full extension [7, 8]

- The coronoid process is the most important stabiliser against posterior and axial dislocation. Furthermore, the anterior bundle of the MCL and the annular ligament insert on the coronoid process [9]
- The sublime tubercle is the medial extension of the coronoid process. The anterior bundle of the MCL inserts at this area [10] Fig. 4.6
- The supinator crest is the lateral distal extension of the sigmoid notch. Besides the supinator muscle the LCL inserts at this area [11]

The proximal ulnashaft is not straight. There are two important angulations that have to be respected during reduction of proximal ulna shaft fractures (Fig. 4.7):

- Proximal ulna dorsal angulation (PUDA)
  From a lateral view the ulnashaft is known to be straight. But the proximal shaft has a dorsal bow with a mean angulation 5.7–8.5° (range 1.7–14.1°). Increasing the PUDA will lead to a decrease of elbow extension [12, 13]

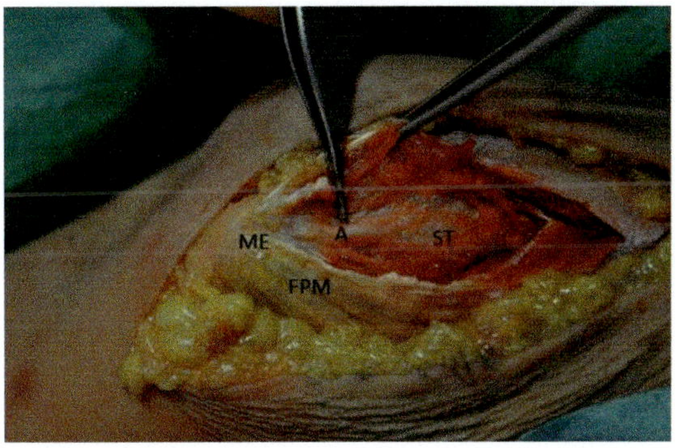

Fig. 4.6 The figure shows the medial aspect of the joint, after longitudinal dissection of the flexor-pronator mass (FPM), originating from the medial epicondyle (ME). Beneath the anterior bundle of the medial collateral ligament (A) is found. It inserts into the sublime tubercle (ST)

- Varus angulation
  The varus angulation of the proximal ulna is also referred to as the "radial bow" or "antero-medial angulation in the proximal third of the ulna". Several studies reported a mean angle of 8.5–17.5° with a range from 2.1–28°. The distance of the apex and the most proximal point of the dorsal surface is a mean 75 mm (59.9–91 mm) [12]

The high interindividual variability of these angles has to be kept in mind during reduction of a proximal shaft fracture. Precontoured proximal ulna locking plates are provided in different lengths but not in different angles. As these plates are designed according to the mean values, the plates most often do not fit perfectly to the ulna due to the wide range of these angles [14]. The surgeon must be aware to adapt these plates to anatomy. Any deviation from perfect anatomy of the ulna shaft may lead to a joint incongruence – especially in Monteggia fractures where the PRUJ is unstable.

Therapeutic Options

Non-operative Treatment

Basically, non-displaced fractures of the olecranon can be treated without surgery. But there is

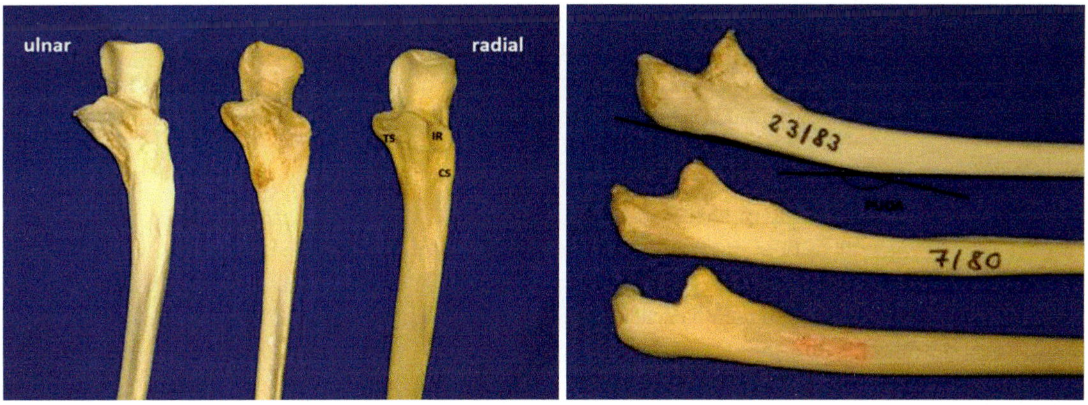

Fig. 4.7 The figure shows the interindividual variety of proximal ulna anatomy. (**a**) (left) The radial bow of the ulna is shown. (*CS* Supinator crest, *TS* Sublime tubercle, *IR* radial incision of the proximal ulna). (**b**) (right) The figure shows the dorsal angulation (PUDA: Proximal ulna dorsal angulation) with its individual variety

no clear consensus on the amount of displacement that is still acceptable for conservative treatment. In accordance to Veillette et al. 2 mm of displacement as a maximum value is supposed for non-operative treatment [15]. If indicated, the elbow is immobilized in a cast in flexion of 80° for 2 weeks with then assisted flexion to 100°. Flexion is increased over the following weeks. For a period of 6 weeks, active extension should be limited to reduce the pull of the triceps muscle. Periodical x-ray controls are mandatory to detect secondary dislocation. It has been reported, that in elderly patients with lower demands, conservative treatment of displaced olecranon fractures can lead to good functional outcomes [16].

Surgical Treatment

Osteosynthesis of the olecranon can be done with tension band wiring, plating, and nailing. Even suture anchor repair has been reported [17]. All treatment methods aim for stable and anatomical reconstruction of the olecranon. As nailing and intramedullary screws do not represent standard treatment, there will be no further discussion.

The procedure is performed from a posterior approach curved around the lateral side of the olecranon tip [18]. The use of a true lateral approach has also been described, but is only rarely used. To get good access to the dorsal aspect of the ulna, the patient should be placed in the lateral decubitus or prone position. Placing the elbow placed in a 90° flexed position is helpful to assist reposition. The decubitus position is also possible with the arm over the chest, but an additional assistant is necessary to stabilize the arm. During the procedure, one has to be aware of the course of the ulnar nerve and its identification is mandatory, when the fracture configuration demands broad dissection. In more simple fractures with adequate soft tissues, the nerve is not necessarily displayed. It is important to respect the soft tissues around the proximal ulna. When significant swelling is present, the timing of the procedure must allow consolidation of the soft tissues.

Due to the different categories of proximal ulna fractures representing different types of injury with different anatomic lesions, the operative treatment protocols differ accordingly. As studies have shown, the decision making by the surgeons whether plating or tension band wiring is performed, depends largely on fracture morphology and comminution. In the following, the treatment protocols are discussed according to the Mayo classification [4].

Mayo Type I A, Mayo Type II A

These fractures represent non-displaced or displaced fractures of the olecranon without comminution. The joint is assessed as stable. Although these fractures can be stabilized with plates, tension band wiring is the most established treatment for these entities. An advantage of this procedure is, that required equipment is limited to 1.6 K-wires and a cerclage wire. It has proven to be a cost effective method, providing consistent clinical results [19]. However, performing the tension band wiring of the ulna is not an easy procedure, as specific tasks have to be achieved on the one hand, and crucial mistakes can be made on the other [20].

As primary aspect, anatomical repositioning of the fracture must be achieved. Therefore it has proven itself to align the dorsal cortices of the fracture fragments, as this will prevent narrowing of the semilunar notch (Fig. 4.5). After cleaning and repositioning of the fracture, the surgeon must place the k-wires in a parallel fashion from proximal to distal, through the medial aspect and the lateral aspect of the olecranon. The recommendations differ, but placing the wires, bicortical seems to give best resistance against retrograde wire pullout. When the k-wires exit the ventral cortex, irritation of the median nerve is unlikely, when protrusion of the wires is less than 1 cm. Perforation of the K-wires on the radial side, nevertheless, may lead to a possible conflict resulting in restricted or impossible forearm rotation (Fig. 4.8). It is essential to take the varus angulation of the proximal ulna into account not to place the wires in a lateral direction and therefore to avoid impingement between hardware and the radius [21]. Besides intraoperative fluoroscopic examination, an accurate intraoperative examination of forearm rotation should

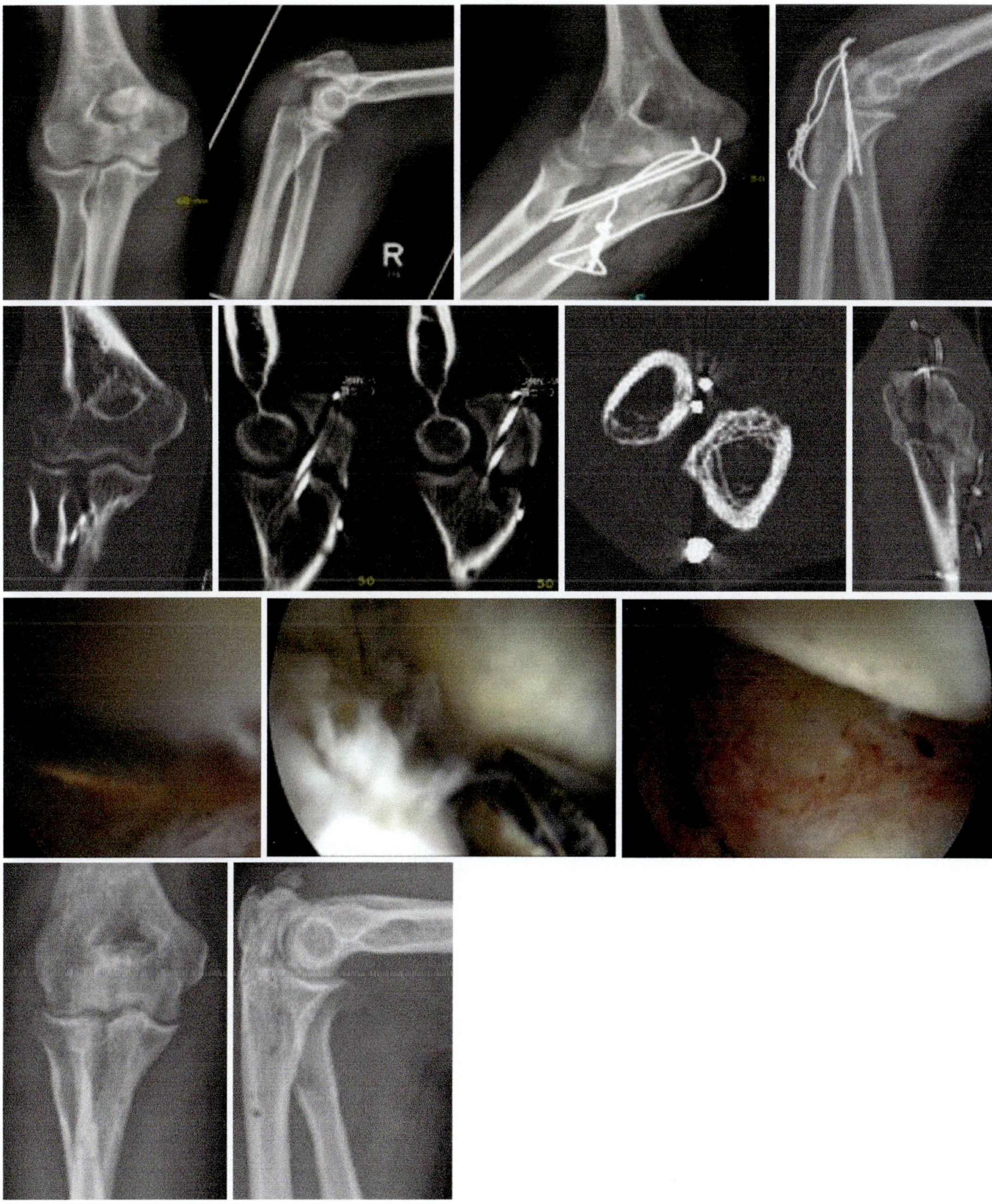

Fig. 4.8 Displaced olecranon fracture stabilized with TBW. Radially perforating K-wires affect the proximal radius leading to complete restriction of forearm rotation. The CT-scan further shows an intraarticular K-wire, poor fracture reduction, an beginning development HO at the PRUJ. The arthroscopy proved intraarticular K-wire placement and severe arthrofibrosis of the PRUJ. As the fracture showed beginning fracture healing a complete metal removal with artrhoscopic realease of the PRUJ was performed resulting in 80° pronation and 60° supination

be performed to ensure free ROM. Perforation of the K-Wires on the ulnar side may harm the ulnar nerve. Bending the proximal ends of the K-wires into the bone offers additional stability and helps hiding the tips within the triceps tendon. The transverse drill hole for the cerclage wire should be place 2–3 cm distal to the fracture line. After the cerclage wire has been placed, we recommend applying a curl on each side, as it facilitates precise adjustment of the compression. To support good woundhealing, closure has to be done thoroughly.

Mayo Type I B, Mayo Type II B, Type III

For comminuted fractures tension band wiring is not adequate in most of the cases. Due to comminution of these fracture types, the surgeon might be misled into expanded dissection of the fracture to improve visualization. However, one has to be aware, that soft tissue dissection on the one hand will decrease to blood supply of the fracture zone, and on the other hand destabilizes the fracture fragments. So indirect repositioning should be preferred with the elbow positioned in an arm holder as 90° flexion supports correct repositioning. Furthermore, it is possible to open the joint at the medial or lateral border of the olecranon, to gain visualization of the fracture zone, and to allow elevation of impacted fragments respectively. It is of primary importance to align the dorsal cortices of the olecranon, to respect the width of the semilunar notch and to reconstruct the sagittal alignment of the olecranon proximal and distal to the bare area. Also, the anatomical alignment in the frontal plane must be achieved because any deviation will transmit dislocating force on the PRUJ, especially in Monteggia-Lesions. Temporary stabilization is realised by longitudinal, bicortical k-wires to facilitate plate mounting or addressing some smaller fragments. When intermediate fragments are present, they should be reposed and fixed if possible (Fig. 4.9). If not possible, however, they can be removed to prevent necrosis of the fragments with generation of loose bodies. Especially in elderly patients, the articular fracture fragments are frequently deep impacted and have to be realigned to the semilunar notch. In these cases, additional bone grafting could be helpful to gain sufficient stabilization.

Different types of plates are available for dorsal stabilization. Especially in multi-fragmented or osteoporotic fractures, angular stable implants are advantageous. Due to the variable anatomy and the thin soft tissue coverage of the proximal

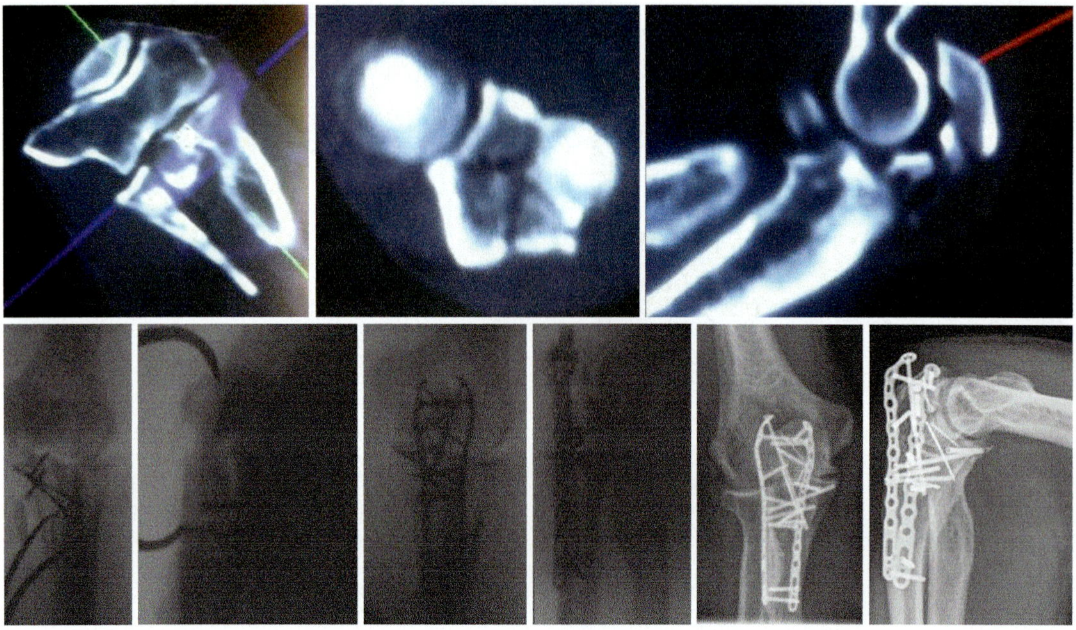

Fig. 4.9 Transolecranon fracture dislocation with a severly comminuted greater sigmoid notch and additional fracture of the sublime tubercule and coronoid process. Multpile small intermediate fragments were fixed with small screws and lost k-wires first before closing the oleranon with perfect shape of the semilunar notch and stabilisation with double plating.The farcture healed uneventfully with a good functional result

ulna, however, the optimum fit of the plates is desirable. Even so, the newer precontoured locking plates have been shown not to fit in the majority of cases, even when skilled recontouring is performed [14].

A new method of plating has been promoted over the last years that offers double plating of the olecranon (Fig. 4.10) [21]. The plates are placed below the anconeus muscle laterally, and belwo the flexor carpi ulnaris muscle medially. A 1 cm

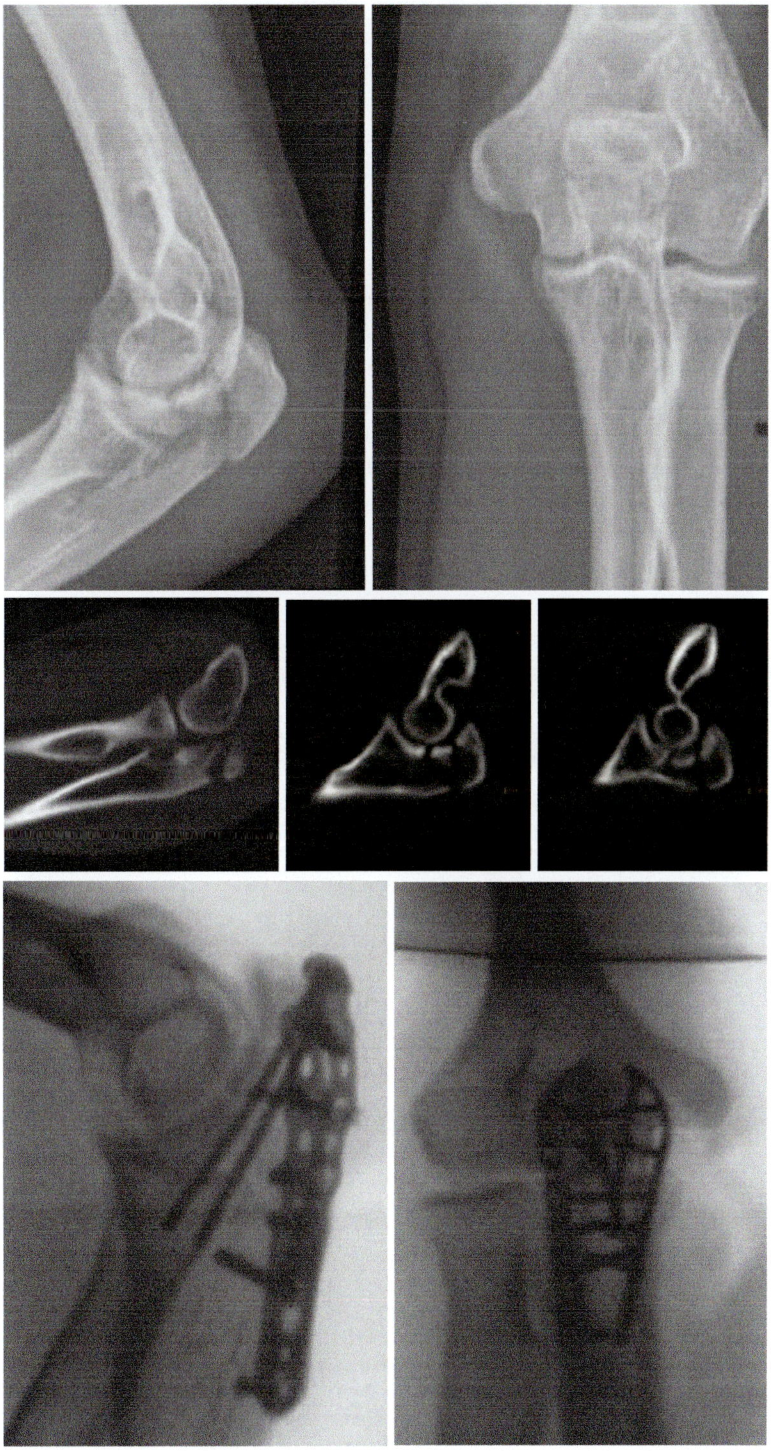

Fig. 4.10 Minimally displaced multifragmentary olecranon fracture in a 30 years old male patient who fell during sports. Fracture was fixed with double plating allowing for early physiotherapy

pocket is generated subperiosteally over the length of the implants. By doing so, soft tissue irritation is brought to a minimum. Thus, hardware removal is less often indicated. Moreover as two plates are involved, up to 14 locking screws can be placed within the bone resulting in a very high primary stability. The proximal screws are placed perpendicular to the force vector of the trizeps pull supporting primary stability.

In Monteggia like lesions, the fractured radial head can be addressed from the posterior approach as well, either through the olecranon fracture or by the Boyd's approach releasing the anconeus and the annular ligament from the lateral olecranon (Fig. 4.11). In that way, a second incision is not necessary. In fracture dislocations, it is necessary to address the soft tissue stabilizers as well by reconstruction of the ligaments with direct suturing, transosseous suturing or with suture anchors. If the fracture affects the sublime tubercle and/or the supinator crest, these structures have to be addressed during osteosynthesis as well to restore the insertion of the AMCL and the LUCL. If primary joint stability is not achieved, a temporary dynamic external fixator may be added.

Postoperative Care

The goal must be an immediate mobilisation of the joint under physiotherapeutic control. After surgery, a plaster cast should be added until wound consolidation. The splint should be applied to the anterior aspect with a swing to the lateral aspect of the upper am to evade the wound and to allow healing. Elevation with supporting lymphatic drainage is often beneficial by reducing swelling of the soft tissues. While surgery has achieved stable fracture fixation we allow passive exercising of full range of motion from the first day. Full weight-bearing is allowed after 3 months. Hardware removal is almost performed for tension band wiring and dorsal locked plating. For the double plating procedure, the removal is necessary in about 40% of the cases.

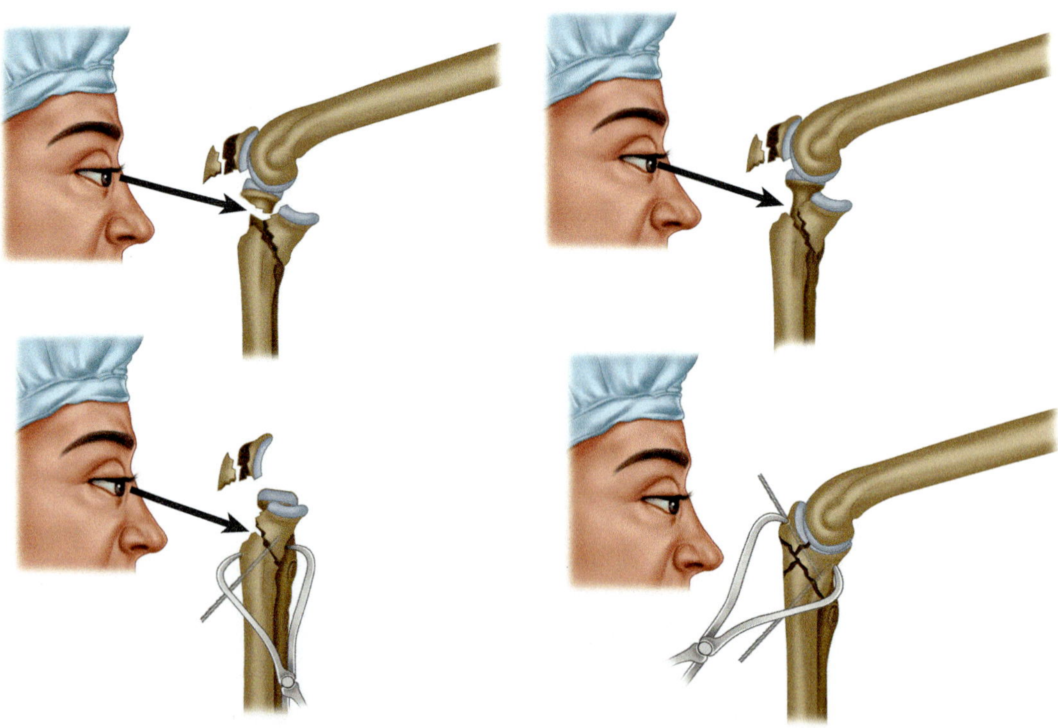

Fig. 4.11 Fracture reduction of the coronoid and radial head through the olecaron facture

Outcomes and Complications

Secondary arthritis after olecranon fractures is low with an incidence of about 7%. Also joint stiffness after surgical treatment of olecranon fractures is less common when compared to other elbow fractures. However, the risk increases with the amount of comminution [22]. In general - following tension band wiring or plating – the outcomes are good to excellent [23]. As the most common complications, malunion, soft tissue irritation by hardware and ulnar neuritis have to be outlined [24]. The risk for complications rises with the severity of the trauma. To our view, soft tissue irritation or symptomatic hardware in general represents the complication with the highest relevance. Hardware removal is usually done 12 months after surgery when bony healing has been confirmed. If soft tissues are comprised by prominent hardware, removal can be performed at an earlier stage. However, fracture healing must be assured. We believe the double plating with a medial and lateral position, hidden under muscles, to be a superior way of fracture treatment, especially when looking at the soft tissue irritation.

References

1. Karlsson MK, Hasserius R, Karlsson C, Besjakov J, Josefsson PO. Fractures of the olecranon: a 15- to 25-year followup of 73 patients. Clin Orthop Relat Res. 2002;403:205–12.
2. Rommens PM, Schneider RU, Reuter M. Functional results after operative treatment of olecranon fractures. Acta Chir Belg. 2004;104(2):191–7.
3. Amis AA, Miller JH. The mechanisms of elbow fractures: an investigation using impact tests in vitro. Injury. 1995;26(3):163–8.
4. Morrey BF. Current concepts in the treatment of fractures of the radial head, the olecranon, and the coronoid. Instr Course Lect. 1995;44:175–85.
5. Colton CL. Fractures of the olecranon in adults: classification and management. Injury. 1973;5(2):121–9.
6. Muller ME, Allgower M, Schneider R, Willenegger H. Comprehensive classification of fractures of long bones. Berlin: Springer; 1991.
7. An KN, Morrey BF, Chao EY. The effect of partial removal of proximal ulna on elbow constraint. Clin Orthop Relat Res. 1986;209:270–9.
8. Bell TH, Ferreira LM, McDonald CP, Johnson JA, King GJ. Contribution of the olecranon to elbow stability: an in vitro biomechanical study. J Bone Joint Surg Am. 2010;92(4):949–57.
9. Morrey BF, An KN. Stability of the elbow: osseous constraints. J Shoulder Elbow Surg. 2005;14(1 Suppl S):174S–8S.
10. Sanchez-Sotelo J, O'Driscoll SW, Morrey BF. Anteromedial fracture of the coronoid process of the ulna. J Shoulder Elbow Surg. 2006;15(5):e5–8.
11. Athwal GS, Faber KJ, King GJ, Elkinson I. Crista supinatoris fractures of the proximal part of the ulna. J Bone Joint Surg Am. 2014;96(4):326–31.
12. Beser CG, Demiryurek D, Ozsoy H, Ercakmak B, Hayran M, Kizilay O, et al. Redefining the proximal ulna anatomy. Surg Radiol Anat. 2014;36(10):1023–31.
13. Rouleau DM, Faber KJ, Athwal GS. The proximal ulna dorsal angulation: a radiographic study. J Shoulder Elbow Surg. 2010;19(1):26–30.
14. Puchwein P, Schildhauer TA, Schoffmann S, Heidari N, Windisch G, Pichler W. Three-dimensional morphometry of the proximal ulna: a comparison to currently used anatomically preshaped ulna plates. J Shoulder Elbow Surg. 2012;21(8):1018–23.
15. Veillette CJ, Steinmann SP. Olecranon fractures. Orthop Clin North Am. 2008;39(2):229–36, vii.
16. Gallucci GL, Piuzzi NS, Slullitel PA, Boretto JG, Alfie VA, Donndorff A, et al. Non-surgical functional treatment for displaced olecranon fractures in the elderly. Bone Joint J. 2014;96-B(4):530–4.
17. Bateman DK, Barlow JD, vanBeek C, Abboud JA. Suture anchor fixation of displaced olecranon fractures in the elderly: a case series and surgical technique. J Shoulder Elbow Surg. 2015;24(7):1090–7.
18. Brolin TJ, Throckmorton T. Olecranon fractures. Hand Clin. 2015;31(4):581–90.
19. Newman SD, Mauffrey C, Krikler S. Olecranon fractures. Injury. 2009;40(6):575–81.
20. Schneider MM, Nowak TE, Bastian L, Katthagen JC, Isenberg J, Rommens PM, et al. Tension band wiring in olecranon fractures: the myth of technical simplicity and osteosynthetical perfection. Int Orthop. 2014;38(4):847–55.
21. Willinger L, Lucke M, Crönlein M, Sandmann GH, Biberthaler P, Siebenlist S. Malpositioned olecranon fracture tension-band wiring results in proximal radioulnar syostosis. Eur J Med Res. 2015;20:87.
22. Erturer RE, Sever C, Sonmez MM, Ozcelik IB, Akman S, Ozturk I. Results of open reduction and plate osteosynthesis in comminuted fracture of the olecranon. J Shoulder Elbow Surg. 2011;20(3):449–54.
23. Tarallo L, Mugnai R, Adani R, Capra F, Zambianchi F, Catani F. Simple and comminuted displaced olecranon fractures: a clinical comparison between tension band wiring and plate fixation techniques. Arch Orthop Trauma Surg. 2014;134(8):1107–14.
24. Matar HE, Ali AA, Buckley S, Garlick NI, Atkinson HD. Surgical interventions for treating fractures of the olecranon in adults. Cochrane Database Syst Rev. 2014;11:CD010144.

Radial Head Fractures

5

Graham J. W. King and Jason A. Strelzow

Epidemiology

Fractures of the radial head are the most common fracture of the elbow, accounting for one-third of all elbow fractures and 3% of all fractures [1]. Two large epidemiological studies demonstrated a mean age of injury of 48 years and a male-female ratio of 2:3. Males are affected at a significantly younger age (37 years) compared to females (52 years) [1]. Fractures of the radial head may occur in isolation or as part of a more complex injury pattern. Isolated elbow injuries more commonly occur with non-displaced fractures. Associated ligamentous injuries or elbow dislocation are commonly seen in the setting of more displaced or comminuted radial head fractures. Bilateral fractures of the radial head and neck are unusual; 1.5% of all radial head fractures [2].

G. J. W. King (✉)
Roth McFarlane Hand and Upper Limb Centre, St. Joseph's Health Centre, Western University, London, ON, Canada
e-mail: graham.king@sjhc.london.on.ca

J. A. Strelzow
Department of Orthopaedic Surgery and Rehabilitation Medicine, University of Chicago, Chicago, IL, USA

Classification

Debate regarding the optimal fracture classification for radial head fractures continues. The Mason classification is arguably the most widely used, however, additional modifications and classification systems exist. Described in 1954 and later modified by others, the Mason classification has been evaluated and found to have satisfactory intra- and inter-observer agreement compared to the AO classification which showed poor to fair reliability [3, 4].

One modification of the Mason classification includes displacement, comminution and associated injuries in an effort to guide treatment (Table 5.1) [5]. None or minimally displaced (<2 mm) fractures are classified as type I; type II are displaced more than 2 mm, type III are comminuted complete articular fractures while type IV includes any fracture associated with a dislocation of the elbow [6] (Fig. 5.1). Recent modifications to this classification system have added associated injuries to the coronoid (c), olecranon (o), distal radio-ulnar joint(d) and ligamentous structures (l) with subscripts [7]. Hotchkiss also modified the Mason classification by uniting the fracture classification with treatment [8].

Unfortunately, the reproducibility of these classifications remains in question. Given the dish shaped nature of the radial head, imaging is problematic, hence defining displacement and fragment size is challenging on plain radiographs [3, 9].

P. Biberthaler et al. (eds.), *Acute Elbow Trauma*, Strategies in Fracture Treatments,
https://doi.org/10.1007/978-3-319-97850-5_5

Distinguishing reconstructable from non-salvageable fractures can be especially problematic pre-operatively, which further questions the utility of these systems [10]. Fundamentally, classification systems may help to broadly categorize radial head injuries, but they do not directly guide treatment.

Symptoms and Diagnostics

A detailed trauma history, medical and surgical history, social history, and hand dominance is required. Specific questioning should focus on the mechanism of injury, location of pain, treatment to date, and the presence of any prior injuries to the elbow. The mechanism of injury should be sought to help determine the possibility of instability or history of dislocation.

Table 5.1 Modified Mason classification as described by Johnston (1962)

Mason classification	Description
I	Non-displaced or fissure fracture
II	Minimally displaced >2 mm or angulated, may or may not be associated with a block to motion
III	Comminuted fracture
IV	Dislocation with concomitant radial head fracture

Examination requires a thorough review of the entire upper extremity. Limb alignment and resting position, status of the soft tissues and neurological examination should be documented in detail. Palpation of the bony prominences of the elbow are methodically examined. Lateral structures including the supracondylar ridge, epicondyle, capitellum, radial tuberosity, radial neck and head are palpated. Corresponding medial structures including the supracondylar ridge, epicondyle, olecranon, proximal ulna and the sublime tubercle are also examined. Palpation along the interosseous membrane and a thorough examination of the distal radio-ulnar joint are performed to rule out associated forearm and wrist injuries.

Elbow motion should be examined with particular attention paid to the presence of a mechanical block to forearm rotation which is an indication for surgical management. If range of motion examination is equivocal or limited due to pain, the joint hematoma can be evacuated with or without the infiltration of intra-articular local anesthetic [11]. Terminal elbow flexion and extension are expected to be lost in the presence

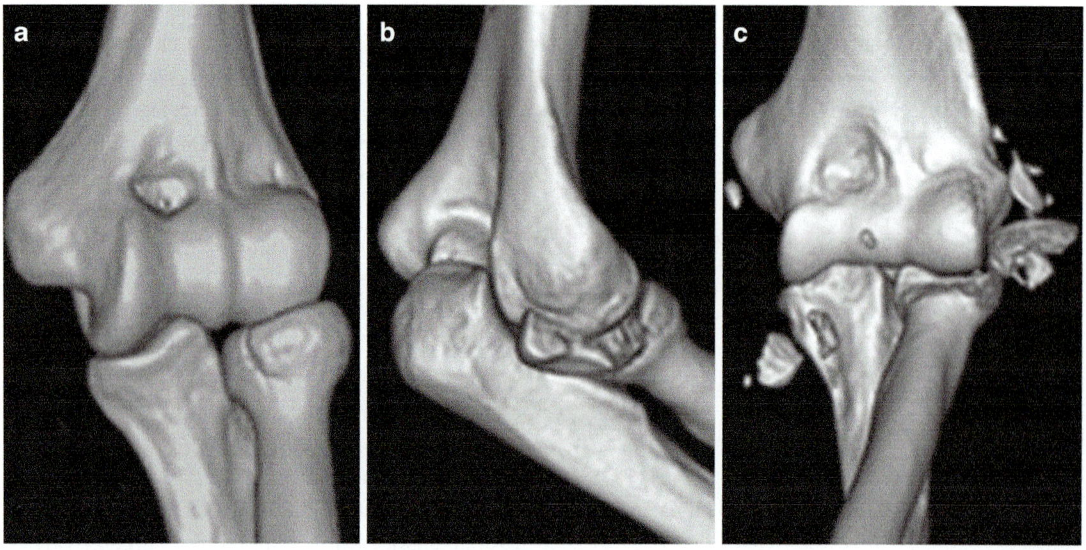

Fig. 5.1 The Mason classification. Type I fractures are none or minimally displaced (**a**). Type II fractures are displaced (**b**). Type III fractures are comminuted (**c**)

of an elbow effusion and should not be mistaken for a mechanical block to motion. An assessment of the ligamentous status of the elbow further delineates a strictly bony injury from more complex osseous-ligamentous injury patterns. Varus, valgus and posterolateral rotatory stability should be documented, however this may be challenging in the acute setting as pain often precludes a reliable examination.

Because assessment of elbow stability is difficult in the acutely traumatized patient, a fluoroscopic examination under anesthesia may be warranted in selected cases. There are a multitude of clinical tests described to assess the collateral ligaments of the elbow [12]. Assessment of the lateral collateral ligament may be clinically examined using the hypersupination test, pivot shift or varus stress test, while the medial collateral structures are evaluated using the valgus stress test and hyperpronation test.

A thorough radiographic examination of the elbow is always required. Anteroposterior, oblique and lateral films should be obtained. Radiographs of the wrist to assess distal radial ulnar joint (DRUJ) injury may also be indicated if wrist pain is present. In the setting of hemarthrosis, it may be difficult to obtain ideal patient positioning for adequate AP radiographs of the elbow. In such circumstances, radiographs in the anteroposterior plane focused first on the distal humerus and subsequently on the forearm provide the necessary views. Subtle fractures may present with a positive 'fat pad sign' signifying elevation of the intra-capsular, extrasynovial fat by a haemarthrosis [13]. The anterior 'fat pad' is a combination of intra-capsular, extra-synovial fat from the coronoid and radial fossa which is typically seen in normal radiographs parallel along the anterior humerus. In contrast, the posterior 'fat pad' consists of the olecranon fat pad and in uninjured elbows is deep within the olecranon fossa and invisible on normal lateral radiographs [13].

Additional elbow views, including the oblique Greenspan view, may help define radial head and neck pathology by avoiding the overlying coronoid [14]. To obtain a Greenspan view, a modified lateral radiograph with 90° of elbow flexion and neutral rotation is performed. The beam is oriented 45° angled towards the radial head travelling in a superior to inferior direction. If there is suspicion for additional axial or varus/valgus instability about the elbow, stress radiographs have been described by Davidson et al. with axial distraction and compression of the forearm by manipulation at the wrist [15]. Intra-operative radiographic assessment of axial instability has more recently been termed the 'radius pull test' [16]. In the setting of radiographic uncertainty or for pre-operative evaluations in the setting of complex injury patterns, computed tomography is helpful [17].

Injury Pattern and Surgery Related Anatomy

Radial head fractures classically result from a fall on an outstretched arm. Forearm position, load characteristics (axial, valgus, varus) and rotational elements are suspected to be responsible for the pattern of concomitant injuries and radial head fracture configuration. The anterolateral portion of the radial head is most frequently fractured [18]. Bone density and volume in the anterolateral quadrant of the head is lowest which may explain this finding [19]. Associated osseous and soft tissue injuries are frequently reported, ranging from 7% to 100% [15, 20]. Disruption of the ligaments of the elbow or forearm are frequently associated with displaced fractures of the radial head, with both the medial and lateral collateral ligament (MCL/LCL) commonly involved [15]. Soft tissue injuries have been documented by magnetic resonance imaging in up to three-quarters of radial head fracture patients, however, the clinical significance of many of these findings may be limited [21]. Undisplaced or minimally displaced fractures are typically isolated injuries without appreciable disruption of the surrounding soft tissue constraints. Associated coronoid fractures are the most common osseous injury [22]. Fracture morphology and location may portend the presence of additional injury [23]. The presence of a large fracture involving the anteromedial quadrant of the radial head was significantly associated with the presence of dislocation. An important but rare associated injury with radial head fracture is the Essex-Lopresti injury. First attributed to Essex-Lopresti in 1951, it entails injury to the interosseous membrane (IOM) and DRUJ creating axial instability between the radius and ulna.

A thorough understanding of elbow anatomy allows the surgeon to contextualize the implications of a radial head fracture. An intricate relationship exists between the articular structures, ligaments and muscles of the elbow to produce the dynamic motion and stability needed for elbow function. Three primary bony articulations, the ulnohumeral, radiocapitellar and proximal radio-ulnar joints (PRUJ) establish a high degree of congruent bony architecture which imparts inherent stability. The radial head has a concave dish shaped articular surface articulating with the spherical capitellum. The radial neck axis is offset from the head to a variable amount [24]. The articulation of the radial head at the radial notch of the ulna has an elliptical shape which generates a cam-effect during rotation producing radial displacement of the radial shaft during pronation [24]. A non-articular 'safe zone' consists of a portion of the radial head which does not articulate with the radial notch of the ulna [25]. The area is described as an arc of 110° in reference to a point 10° above the midpoint of the lateral radial head with the forearm in neutral rotation. This zone can also be localized by its more rounded appearance compared to the flatter articulating surface, thinner cartilage with a colour difference, and by visualizing an arc between Lister's tubercle and the radial styloid [26].

Radial head blood supply has two main sources: intraosseous and extraosseous. The extra osseous blood supply is from dual sources. A single branch off the radial recurrent artery feeds the head directly, while the interosseous recurrent and the radial artery provide additional vasculature through insertions penetrating the capsule at the radial neck [27]. Careful preservation of the periosteal attachments is important to optimize vascularity of fracture fragments.

The radial head has three main roles in elbow stability; axial stability, varus/posterolateral rotatory instability, and as a secondary restraint for valgus stability [28].

Considerable force is transmitted through the radio-capitellar joint during upper extremity activities [29]. Proximal migration of the radius is primarily restrained by the radial head articulation with the capitellum. Secondary longitudinal stability is imparted through soft tissue structures including the interosseous ligament and the DRUJ. Axial stability and loading across the radio-capitellar joint changes with forearm positioning. Approximately 60% of the force applied to the arm is transmitted through the radiocapitellar joint [30]. This force transmission varies dependent on the amount of elbow flexion and extension [31]. Maximal force across the radiocapitellar joint occurs during pronation between zero and 30° of elbow flexion with decreasing force transmission as flexion increases [32].

The radial head acts as a secondary valgus stabilizer [31, 33]. The MCL is the primary restraint to valgus force. The radial head provides secondary elbow stability when the collateral ligament structures and soft tissues of the forearm (distal radial ulnar joint, triangular fibrocartilage or interosseous membrane) are intact. Biomechanical data suggests that the radial head contributes 24% to varus-valgus laxity if excised [34]. The radial head is of critical importance when primary stabilizers are disrupted [34]. The radial head alters the MCL lever arm load by changing the varus/valgus rotational plane, which suggests that retention of the radial head is important for long term elbow stability [33]. The radial head may also confer varus stability to the elbow through tensioning of the lateral ligament [35].

Radial head fractures affecting the articular surface area of the radiocapitellar joint have importance when considering overall stability of the elbow. A biomechanical study found a direct relationship between radial head fracture size and radiocapitellar stability [36]. Radial head fractures involving more than one-third of the articular surface were determined to significantly decrease radiocapitellar stability [36]. Fracture fragment size is of particular importance with additional compromise to the adjacent supports including the

MCL, LCL, coronoid, and capitellum, as may be seen in simple or complex elbow dislocations and terrible triad injury patterns. Despite these biomechanical studies, limited clinical data exists to direct definitive clinical practice.

An understanding of the fracture personality, including the amount of fracture displacement, surface area involved, and comminution may serve as an early identifier of more complex injury patterns necessitating additional work up [15].

Therapeutic Options

Radial head fracture management encompasses both operative and non-operative treatment options. A thorough understanding of the osseous injuries and concomitant soft tissue trauma is critical to the appropriate selection of treatment modalities. Treatment plans should consider patient specific factors (bone quality, age, activity demands), surgeon competence, equipment availability and injury pattern.

Non-operative Treatment

Controversy remains regarding which radial head fractures should be treated non-operatively. Established indications include; non-displaced fractures (Mason Type I) and displaced fractures without a block to motion (Mason Type II). Consensus regarding the size of fracture fragment and the amount of displacement has not been established. Biomechanical studies would suggest that fractures involving less than 25% and potentially up to a third of the articular surface do not result in substantial change to joint mechanics [36]. This is corroborated by a number of clinical studies documenting successful non-operative treatment of fractures involving less than 25% or 2 mm of depression at the radial head [5]. In addition, a number of studies have demonstrated successful non-operative management of more displaced fractures (Mason II and III) without rotational block [37, 38].

Non-operative management involves a short period of immobilization, typically less than one week, dictated by the patients comfort. Early motion is paramount to prevent stiffness and begins with active pronation, supination, flexion and extension exercises [39]. The patient should continue to utilize a collar and cuff when at rest or ambulating to prevent unintentional loading as well as to alert others to their injury. The collar and cuff is generally discontinued 4 weeks post injury. Scheduled follow-up should include a 10–14 day repeat radiograph to assess for maintenance of fracture reduction/position and to ensure their range of motion is progressing. Shulman et al. suggested we may be over-treating isolated Type I injuries finding no radiographic or physical exam findings that changed management at any time point beyond the primary visit [40]. Elbow motion should recover to near full by approximately 6 weeks. Therapy referral may be required if persistent stiffness exists at the 6 week follow-up visit.

Surgical Treatment (Including Radial Head Arthroplasty)

The only current surgical indication which has been established is a radial head fracture which is impeding motion. Radial head fracture surgery may also be considered in the setting of complex elbow or forearm instability requiring stabilization. Surgical treatment options include: radial head fragment excision, complete head excision, open reduction and internal fixation as well as radial head arthroplasty (Fig. 5.2). Regardless of the technique, surgical exposure of the fracture requires a careful understanding of the anatomy to optimize visualization and minimize complications.

Surgical Approaches

Patient positioning is either in the supine or lateral position. The supine position provides a familiar and easy protocol for the surgical team and anesthesia. The affected arm is positioned across the chest with a sandbag or IV bag bolster which can be positioned underneath the ipsilateral scapula to support the arm. Alternatively a hand table can be employed. Access to the medial and lateral elbow can be gained with this positioning. It is important

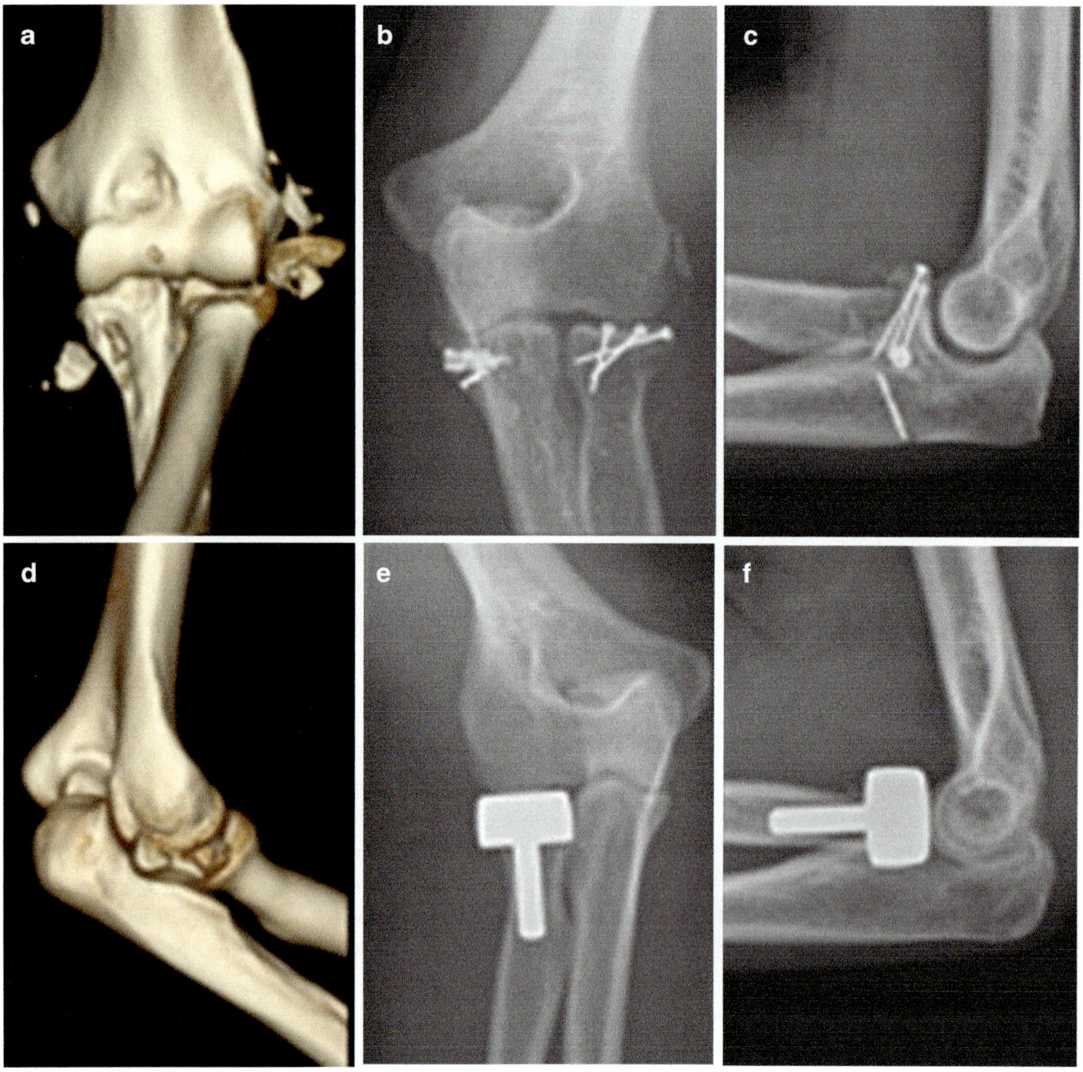

Fig. 5.2 ORIF & Radial Head Arthroplasty for radial head fractures. (**a**) 3-D Computer Tomography (CT) demonstrates a Mason Type 3 Radial head fracture with associated bony and ligamentous injury. (**b**, **c**) Post-operative films following open reduction and internal fixation (ORIF). (**d**) 3D-CT of a Mason Type 2 Radial head fracture. (**e**, **f**) Post-operative films following successful radial head arthroplasty with a loose-polished stemmed arthroplasty

to note pre-operative shoulder range of motion however, as patients with limited external rotation may not be able to deliver the medial elbow structures into a position amenable for the surgeon when using an arm table. If the patient is in the lateral decubitus position, a bolster can hold the affected arm. A sterile tourniquet is used.

One of two possible skin incisions may be utilized; the choice of which is dictated by the presence of additional injuries that require surgical management. A lateral based incision increases the risk to cutaneous crossing nerves and potentially creates skin bridge complications if additional procedures are requiring a posterior or medial incision. The posterior incision may have improved cosmesis and allow for circumferential access to the deeper structures, but may increase the risk of flap necrosis and seroma [41].

If a posterior incision is utilized and extensive skin flaps are raised, using a drain post-operatively for 24 h should be considered. Additionally, dead space beneath the skin flaps should be closed using buried sutures holding the fascia to the subcutaneous tissue.

The lateral skin incision is planned to correspond to the deeper inter-muscular surgical interval. The posterior skin incision begins proximal to the olecranon tip. The incision is carried distally centered on the triceps and just lateral to the olecranon to end along the subcutaneous border of the ulna. The triceps and forearm fascia are preserved while full thickness flaps are elevated. A lateral flap is mobilized to expose the lateral elbow and extensor fascia. Identification and protection of the ulnar nerve is performed if medial sided access is required.

A number of variations of the lateral approach to the elbow exist. Competence of the LCL and osseous structures of interest dictate the ideal plane for deep dissection. Importantly, the forearm should be kept fully pronated during lateral approaches to the radial head to displace the posterior interosseous nerve away from the area of dissection within the supinator musculature [42]. The Kocher approach utilizes the interval between the extensor carpi ulnaris and the anconeus [43]. A fat stripe often helps define the interval allowing the surgeon to incise along this interval from the lateral epicondyle. The capsule is encountered and the extensor carpi ulnaris is elevated anteriorly to incise the capsule above the LUCL. The original Kocher description performed a capsular incision directly through the intermuscular interval which released the LUCL. This approach can be extended proximally and distally and provides excellent access to the LCL should reconstruction or reattachment be required. Distal exposure requires care as the posterior interosseous nerve will be encountered ~4–8 cm distal to the articular surface of the radial head [42]. In the setting of uninjured lateral ligaments, however, the approach limits anterior radial head exposure and risks injury to the ligamentous structures potentially destabilizing the elbow.

The Kaplan approach, by comparison, overcomes the shortcomings of the Kocher approach, limiting risk to the LUCL and providing excellent radial head exposure [44]. Direct palpation of the anterior margin of the radial head provides a landmark for the skin incision. An intermuscular plane between the extensor digitorum communis (EDC) and the extensor carpi radialis longus/brevis (ECRB/L) is used. Deep dissection involves an incision splitting the lateral annular ligament. The Kaplan approach is not extensile distally and does not allow access to the LUCL for repair without additional release of the common extensor tendons [45].

More recently, the common extensor tendon splitting approach, has been demonstrated to be superior to the Kocher for radial head exposure [46]. The common extensor split allows complete visualization of the anterior half of the radial head compared to only 68% of the head utilizing the Kocher approach. This technique also minimizes the soft tissue dissection necessary and thereby reduces the possibility of iatrogenic LUCL injury. The common extensor split can be accessed through either a lateral or posterior skin incision. The common extensor tendon is identified and split centrally from its origin at the lateral epicondyle to approximately 25 mm distal to the radiocapitellar joint [46]. Once through the tendon and capsule, the radial collateral and annular ligament are split inline with the incision at the capitellar equator to prevent LUCL injury. This approach can be extended proximally by detaching the anterior EDC tendon and ECRB off the lateral epicondyle and supracondylar ridge. A cuff of tissue should be left on the humerus to facilitate interval closure.

Closure begins with assessment of the collateral ligament and extensor muscle origins. If the LUCL is intact and the elbow is deemed stable closure of the anterior half of the collateral ligament along with the annular ligament can be completed with absorbable suture in an interrupted fashion so long as the posterior half of the ligament is intact. Care should be taken to ensure closure of this layer does not over tighten and constrain the elbow. If the elbow is unstable with complete detachment of the LCL; repair is indicated. The LCL insertion site at the isometric axis of the elbow is localized at the centre of the circle formed by the capitellum. This repair can be performed with heavy non-absorbable suture using various techniques (transosseous tunnels, suture anchors or endo-button). Likewise, the extensor musculature is similarly repaired. Range of motion and stability should be checked at the completion of the deep soft tissue closure. An intra-operative assessment of a stable arc should be documented to guide rehabilitation post-operatively.

Fragment Excision

Indications for fragment excision include: a small (<25%) fracture fragment resulting in a mechanical block to motion. Larger fragments should undergo open reduction and internal fixation if possible. Fractures greater than 25% of the articular surface should not be excised due to the well documented resulting instability [36]. Small case studies have detailed less favourable outcomes with fragment excision when compared to fixation [47]. Fragment excision can be performed using an open approach as described above or arthroscopically using standard arthroscopy techniques.

Head Excision

Radial head excision was common practice historically, however, with the rise of newer fixation strategies and arthroplasty options its role in fracture management has come under increasing scrutiny. Indications for isolated radial head excision include: comminuted or displaced fractures blocking motion and as a delayed salvage procedure for the management of complications resulting from non-operative treatment [48]. Excision of the radial head *should only be considered* in stable elbows without concomitant soft tissue or osseous injuries or dislocation. Therefore, the number of suitable cases for this treatment modality is likely small given the frequency of associated injuries with more severe fractures. Excision is less technically demanding when compared to arthroplasty or open reduction and internal fixation (ORIF) [49]. Critical to the success of this procedure is restoration of the soft tissue constraints to the elbow following excision of the radial head. Careful preservation of the LUCL is required.

Resection of the radial head may employ an open or arthroscopic technique [50]. Arthroscopic excision uses standard elbow arthroscopy principles and portals [51]. Arthroscopy has a theoretical advantage by minimizing additional ligamentous and capsular trauma compared to open arthrotomy. Recent small series have documented the safe and successful excision of the radial head without complications [52]. That said, experience with arthroscopy of the elbow is recommended before attempting this more advanced arthroscopic technique.

Intra-operative stress radiographs are required to document the absence of valgus, varus or posterolateral rotatory instability [15]. The "radius pull test" can help establish the presence or absence of longitudinal instability [16]. To perform the "pull test' intra-operatively the patients forearm is placed flat on the table in neutral rotation. A longitudinally applied force (approximately 20lbs) is placed on the proximal radius while radiographic evaluation measures changes in ulnar variance prior to, during and with release of the applied traction [16]. A change in variance of equal to or more than 3 mm is suggestive of an IOM injury and more than 6 mm suggests all longitudinal stabilizers are lost. Such instability is considered a contra-indication to isolated radial head excision.

Open Reduction and Internal Fixation (ORIF)

Evidence based guidance regarding the ideal role of open reduction and internal fixation for radial head fractures is lacking. Often the ability to judge appropriateness of repair can only be established intra-operatively [10]. Proposed indications include: fractures involving greater than one-third of the radial head with displacement greater than 2 mm, and any fractures with a mechanical block to motion [53]. Of these only the mechanical block to motion is an absolute indication for surgery. Goals of ORIF should focus on restoration of articular congruity and stability about the elbow. Fixation should allow for early mobilization which has been shown to be associated with improved outcomes [54]. If a strong, stable construct is not attainable at the time of surgery consideration should be given to radial head excision or arthroplasty. Secondary or revision fixation is associated with poorer clinical and surgical outcomes [55]. Ring et al. reported higher complications and poorer outcomes when performing ORIF of more than three fragments [53].

Open reduction and surgical fixation is currently the standard of care. Arthroscopic assisted techniques have been described, however their indications and efficacy remain unclear [56]. Potential advantages are the percutaneous nature of the technique and improved visualization. Concerns regarding fluid extravasation, fracture site bleeding compromising arthroscopic clarity, neurologic injury as well as the technically demanding nature of arthroscopic fixation have precluded widespread adoption of this technique [57].

Fixation can be achieved with bio-absorbable pins, threaded k-wires, headless screws, standard screws or plates. Successful results have been reported with all these modalities [54]. Hardware placement at the articular margin takes advantage of stronger bone but requires countersinking to prevent radial notch impingement. Plate fixation, often required for radial neck fractures with comminution, must be placed in the non-articular 'safe zone' (Fig. 5.3). Evidence from biomechanical studies suggest fixed angle plates provide a superior construct compared to conventional T-plating [58]. Cross-cannulated screw fixation is preferred over plate fixation of non-comminuted neck fractures as the incidence of rotational stiffness is lower [59, 60]. Pre-contoured locking plates are now available which simplifies fixation of more comminuted fractures.

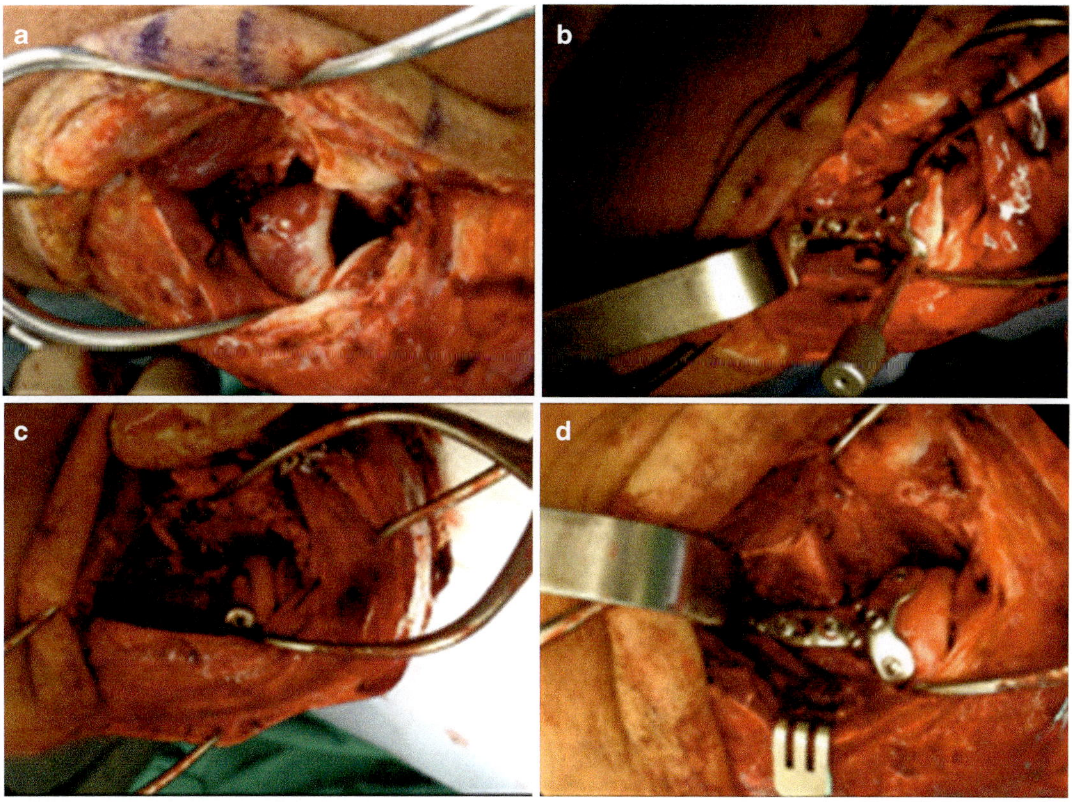

Fig. 5.3 Hardware placement in the "safe zone" is paramount. Identification of the safe zone with rotation of the forearm (**a**). Positioning of the plate within the non-articular portion of the radial head (**b**). Examination of the hardware position to ensure no impingement in supination (**c**) and pronation (**d**)

Careful evaluation for concomitant chondral injuries, fractures and ligament disruption when performing ORIF is essential to ensure an optimal outcome [21]. Osteocartilagenous injuries to the capitellum have been documented in up to 29% of patients [61]. Clinically relevant capitellar osteochondral lesions were reported with a 2% incidence by Van Riet et al. [20]. Caputo et al. (2006) documented a series of cases of minimally displaced fractures with posterolateral capitellar chondral injuries that blocked reduction of the radial head fractures [62]. Capitellar bone bruising was seen in 96% of patients imaged with MRI following radial head fractures [61]. The high incidence of capitellar injury likely results from the compressive load of the radial head against the convex capitellum surface. Itamura et al. also reported up to 92% of patients had associated loose bodies following displaced or comminuted radial head fractures [61].

Arthroplasty

Radial head arthroplasty allows surgical management of displaced, comminuted fractures that are not amenable to anatomic reduction and fixation. Arthroplasty techniques are particularly helpful in the setting of concomitant soft tissue injury allowing for the reliable restoration of elbow stability [63]. Radial head arthroplasty is contraindicated for repairable fractures or in patients with active infection. A relative contraindication is the presence of capitellar arthrosis or severe concomitant chondral injuries.

Surgical approaches for arthroplasty vary, but most commonly a common extensor split or a Kocher interval are utilized dependent on associated ligamentous injuries as outlined previously.

The radial head fragments are removed and reassembled to ensure complete removal. Additional radial neck resection is then done according to the system used, minimizing the resection to create a smooth and perpendicular cut for seating of the prosthetic replacement. Additional chondral and osseous injuries to the surrounding tissue can then be evaluated and managed as appropriate. Fixation of concomitant coronoid fractures should be performed prior to radial head replacement as the prosthesis obstructs the view of the coronoid.

Most current generation modular metallic prostheses allow multiple sizing options overcoming many of the complications previously associated with early generation mono block designs.

Available implant designs include rigidly fixed stems and intentionally loose polished stems. The implants may have bipolar or monopolar articulations. Design features include axisymmetric circular implants as well as nonaxisymmetric elliptical designs. The optimal radial head prosthetic design remains a topic of contention. Shannon et al. examined conventional axisymmetric, elliptical and patient-specific fixed stem implants and compared these to native radial heads [64]. No biomechanical advantage was noted between implant designs, however, all fixed stemmed implant designs altered kinematic motion compared to the native head. No clinical data currently supports the superiority of monopolar over bipolar designs, however our preference is a smooth stem monopolar design [65]. Proposed advantages of bipolar implants are improved radiocapitellar tracking and contact area with a possible decrease in contact pressures. These theoretical advantages come at a potential risk of polyethylene induced osteolysis, reduced elbow and forearm stability, and head-neck dissociation [66, 67].

Correct implant sizing is critical to a successful arthroplasty regardless of the implant design. Prosthesis sizing includes diameter and height sizing. Preoperative templating based on the unaffected 'normal' radial head provides a rough evaluation of expected size. This technique is particularly useful in the setting of prior radial head excision. Intra-operative measurement of the reassembled excised fragments allows for a more accurate assessment of implant size. Minimum head diameter provides the most accurate assessment of size; especially in the setting of comminution of the radial head template [68]. If the templated size is between available implant diameters the smaller size should be selected.

Establishing the correct radial head height is imperative. Measuring the height of the excised radial head is most reliable. Numerous techniques are reported in the literature and can be combined to ensure the appropriate selection of implant size. In the absence of a lateral or interosseous ligament injury the space between the capitellum and radial neck can be used. If a lateral ligament injury is present, and it commonly is, the height of the implant should be at the level of the radial notch about 2 mm distal to the coronoid [69]. Visual inspection of the lateral ulnohumeral joint space during implant positioning was investigated by Athwal et al. and found to be reliable; however a dental mirror is required [70]. They found the use of fluoroscopy to assess for parallel medial and lateral ulnohumeral joint space was insensitive in predicting overstuffing. Notable widening was not appreciated until more than 6 mm of overstuffing was present. Elbow range of motion may also help assess appropriate implant size. Loss of motion in flexion can imply overstuffed lateral components as the radiocapitellar gap tightens in flexion [71]. Work by Grewal et al. [72] suggested that modular prostheses may reduce the frequency of overstuffing more commonly seen in the past with monoblock components.

Following the selection of the radial head diameter and height reaming of the medullary canal is performed. The medullary canal is identified using a blunt tipped instrument (snap, canal finder or entry reamer). Hand reaming is completed until cortical contact is encountered. Stem size is then selected dependent on the system utilized. Some stems are smooth and deliberately placed 1 mm smaller than the reamer size; others are uncemented and require a tight press fit to achieve reliable osseointegration Trial components should be inserted to assess for implant height, diameter, congruency and tracking both visually as well as fluoroscopically.

Postoperative Care

Postoperative care is dictated by elbow stability, intra-operative findings and definitive treatment modality. Associated injuries may delay or change post-operative protocols, therefore, no single ideal rehabilitation protocol exists. Standard post-operative protocols for antibiotic prophylaxis are utilized with 24 h of continued peri-operative antibiotics. Heterotopic ossification (HO) prophylaxis can be used in select patients without contra-indications to anti-inflammatory medications (elderly, history of gastric ulcer, kidney disease, asthma and known allergy). Indomethacin 25 mg three times per day for 3 weeks duration can be utilized. Post-operative HO formation can occur in a significant number of radial head fractures ranging from 3% up to 43% dependent on injury severity and treatment modality [73]. It is not known if indomethacin is effective at reducing the frequency of heterotopic ossification.

Rehabilitation following radial head fracture surgery should be individualized according to injury pattern. Immediate immobilization and elevation post-operatively for a short period of 24–48 h helps facilitate swelling and edema control as well as wound healing.

In stable elbows the arm may be splinted in extension using an anterior slab to minimize flexion contractures and decrease posterior wound tension. Early active motion should be initiated within a few days post-operatively, soft tissues permitting. An early extension program is begun with static progressive splinting at nighttime. Extension splinting is utilized for 12 weeks and adjusted as required while extension improves.

If ligamentous status was tenuous, a repair was performed or instability was documented at the completion of the procedure a ligament protective program is initiated. The elbow is splinted at 60–90° of flexion with the forearm rotated in the optimal position for stability. The established intra-operative safe arc guides rehabilitation. The position of safety dictates the position of the forearm during extension exercises. Lateral ligament injured elbows should be extended with the forearm in pronation. Conversely, elbows with medial ligamentous instability should be extended in supination. Elbows with combined medial and lateral ligament injuries are extended with the forearm in neutral rotation. Forearm rotation is permitted at 90° of flexion or greater as instability is more common with the elbow in extension. When not performing therapy the arm is protected in a resting splint in 90° of flexion and in a safe position of forearm rotation for 3–6 weeks. Timing to wean the resting splint should be individualized to the patient based on radiographic and clinical re-assessment which guides ongoing therapy. If a drop sign or other additional radiographic signs of instability are present, or the fracture fixation is tenuous an overhead protocol can be employed [74]. This modality enables the compressive force of gravity to concentrically reduce the joint, limiting hinging at the articular surface [75]. This is particularly useful prior to the return of physiologic dynamic stabilization from the peri-articular musculature. Extension splinting and passive stretching are generally not implemented until 6 weeks post-operatively due to concerns about heterotopic ossification. Strengthening programs are begun once fracture healing is assured and any soft tissue injury has adequately recovered. Typically strengthening is not begun until at least 8 weeks post-operatively.

Outcomes and Complications

Non-operative Outcomes

Radial head fractures that are undisplaced and fractures with 2–5 mm displacement without a block to rotation treated non-operatively have predominantly favourable outcomes. Delayed radial head resection can be employed if the early outcomes are unacceptable [39, 40, 76–79]. Most long term outcome studies have demonstrated good to excellent results in fractures of less than one-third of the radial head without bony block or clicking during rotation. Persistent radiological deformity is consistently reported with an average loss of 10° of extension but no correlation between x-ray findings and degree of deformity has been reported [5, 76]. A 2012 retrospective study from Edinburgh found socioeconomic factors predicted patient outcomes. Equivalent outcomes were noted between operative and non-operative treatment modalities for all fracture types [80]. More recently a small prospective study of 94 patients documented no difference between immobilization or physiotherapy and clinical outcome [79]. Duckworth et al. reported good or excellent outcomes at 10 year follow-up of 57 Mason Type I and 43 Mason Type II fractures rated by the Disabilities of the Arm, Shoulder and Hand score (DASH) and Oxford Elbow Score [78]. These more recent studies provide compelling evidence that mid- and long-term outcomes following appropriately selected isolated undisplaced and non-comminuted displaced fractures without a mechanical block to motion can be managed non-operatively.

Non-operative Complications

Displacement of previously undisplaced fractures with early motion has been reported [37]. Additional complications include non-union, post-traumatic arthritis and painful malunion [76]. These complications can be managed with late surgical treatments including, radial head excision, osteotomy, fragment excision or arthroplasty [81].

Radial Head Excision Outcomes

Numerous studies support good to excellent short and long term outcomes in patients with fractures not amenable to open reduction internal fixation treated by open radial head excision [48]. These studies demonstrate consistently poor radiological results with proximal migration of the radius, increased carrying angle, increased DRUJ abnormalities and asymptomatic osteoarthritic changes in both the elbow and wrist [82]. Other studies have reported less success [83–85]. Arthroscopic radial head excision has also been demonstrated to improve pain and mechanical symptoms [86]. Regardless of surgical technique clinical elbow motion reported in the literature following radial head excision is typically in a functional range with mild losses of motion.

Radial Head Excision Complications

There are numerous complications reported following radial head excision including; arthritis at the DRUJ and elbow, proximal migration of the radius with ulnar impaction syndrome, instability, increased carrying angle, restriction of elbow/forearm motion, ulnar neuritis and periarticular heterotrophic ossification [82]. Despite several studies stating that these complications were of little functional impact for most patients, for others elbow pain and restricted motion can be problematic. Two series highlight disability associated with radial head excision in the setting of trauma, reporting surgical management of symptomatic missed Essex-Lopresti injuries [84]. Mild loss of supination and extension is common but are generally compatible with satisfactory clinical outcomes [50]. Posterolateral elbow instability after radial head excision is a well-recognized complication occurring in up to 17 percent of patients [87]. Radial head excision in patients with ligamentous injury leads to gross instability with a functionally disabled and painful elbow [83, 85]. Timing of excision is also controversial due to concerns regarding heterotopic ossification (HO). Head injury and associated elbow dislocation are established risk factors associated with HO [88]. Proponents of early (within 24 h) and delayed excision (10 days) exist, however, no definitive guidelines for the optimal timing of radial head excision are available [89].

Open Reduction and Internal Fixation Outcomes

Results from open reduction and internal fixation of displaced radial head fractures suggest good to excellent outcomes in 85–90% of patients [55]. Increasing radial head comminution negatively correlates with final outcome [47]. Functional motion is typically restored in most patients with a modest loss of terminal range [54]. Results of ORIF have been reported to be superior to radial head excision, however, randomized clinical trials are not available [90]. A study by Zarattini et al. [91] demonstrated substantial improvements in the ORIF group compared to the radial head excision group. Overall, the ORIF patients reported less residual pain, reduced risk of subluxation, lower incidence of radiocapitellar arthrosis, greater ROM and improved functional scores [90]. The efficacy of ORIF in isolated partial articular displaced (2–5 mm) radial head fractures has recently been challenged [92]. Outcomes of non-operative and ORIF treatment groups were equivalent. Treatment of both complex (associated fractures, dislocation or soft tissue injury) and isolated radial head injuries may have similar patient reported outcomes and major complications [92, 93]. Comparing ORIF and arthroplasty Watters et al. demonstrated no substantial functional differences in patients with terrible triad injuries, however, arthroplasty significantly improved elbow stability between cohorts [94]. A similar study by Leigh et al. (2012) refuted this finding demonstrating equivalent stability at short-term follow up [95]. Randomized clinical trials comparing treatment methods are needed.

Open Reduction and Internal Fixation Complications

Non-union, avascular necrosis, neurologic injury, recalcitrant pain, stiffness hardware failure and ectopic ossification are potential complications from operative fixation [10]. Combined interruption to the interosseous and extra-osseous blood supply of fracture fragments likely represents the key aetiology for avascular necrosis and non-union of the head/neck [27]. Heterotopic ossification of the post traumatic elbow can be problematic particularly with surgically managed injuries (Fig. 5.4). A recent study documented a 43% rate of HO in surgically treated fracture-dislocations about the elbow with no relationship documented between patient demographics,

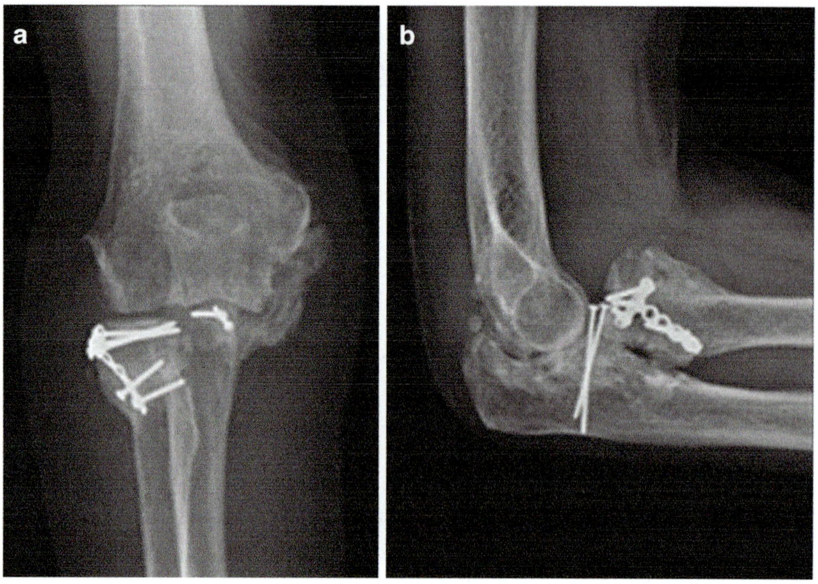

Fig. 5.4 Complications of open reduction and internal fixation of complex radial head trauma. Visible malunion, incongruence of the ulno-humeral joint and radiocapitellar joint with heterotypic ossification (**a**). Articular penetration of the hardware is also appreciated on the lateral xrays (**b**)

co-morbidities, type of surgical strategy, management of associated injuries or time to surgery [96]. Only multiple attempted reductions was found to be associated with HO risk. Posterior interosseous nerve injury has been reported to occur at an incidence of between 1% and 10% [54].

Radial Head Arthroplasty Outcomes

Short and medium term outcomes for metallic radial head replacement have been good or excellent in most series [65]. Functional outcomes, reported by Moro et al. of 25 cases of non-salvageable radial head fractures undergoing metallic radial head arthroplasty reported 17 good or excellent outcomes, with 5 fair and 3 poor at 39 months of follow-up [97]. Unfortunately, there remains a paucity of long-term outcome data. Harrington et al. [65] and others have demonstrated attainment of excellent or good outcomes in 80% of patients, however, others have reported less favourable mid-term follow-up [98]. Implant design and concomitant injuries may explain the difference in outcome between series. Metal radial head replacement restored stability during treatment of fractures in combination with concomitant soft tissue and bony injury [63]. Range of motion was functional in most patients with minor loss of flexion, extension and forearm rotation. In two randomized controlled trials arthroplasty significantly outperformed open reduction and internal fixation achieving higher clinical scores with significantly lower complication rates [98, 99].

Radial Head Arthroplasty Complications

A number of complications are reported in the literature including: radial neck osteolysis, capitellar erosion, stiffness, instability, heterotopic ossification and neurologic injury [71]. Overstuffing the radiocapitellar joint is suggested as the cause of many of the complications associated with arthroplasty. Arthritic changes have been reported in 19% of patients with radial head replacements and would be expected to increase with longer term follow-up [72]. Findings of extensive arthritic change post-operatively from radial head arthroplasty may result from the initial trauma or may be due to secondary changes in the ulnohumeral kinematics and abnormal stresses at the cartilaginous surfaces [100]. Inappropriate radial prosthesis size may be at least partly responsible for these changes, as was

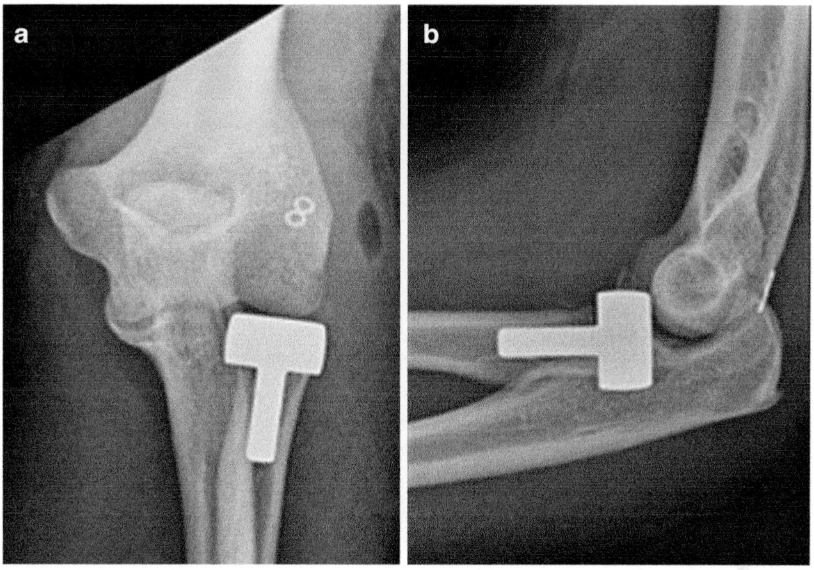

Fig. 5.5 (**a**) AP radiograph after LCL repair and radial head arthroplasty demonstrates residual posterolateral instability. (**b**) Subluxation is better appreciated on the lateral radiographs

suggested by Van Glabbeek et al. demonstrating the importance of correct component sizing [100]. Revision or removal rates for radial head replacement have been variable ranging from 0 to 28% at a mean of 6.7 years after injury [78, 101]. The majority of these patients underwent revision during the first year post-operatively. Revision procedures included: ulnar nerve decompression/transposition, arthrolysis for persistent stiffness, loosening, pain and inappropriate prosthesis size [101]. Flinkkilä et al. (2012) reported a 24% revision rate in patients with two designs of press-fit stems; most of these being early failures [102]. Revision has been less commonly reported in implants using a smooth stem [72, 97, 103]. Failure to restore the lateral ligamentous stability following bipolar arthroplasty of the radial head may be associated with higher complication rates [104]. Residual instability after radial head arthroplasty likely represents additional pathology not addressed during the index procedure (Fig. 5.5).

References

1. Kaas L, van Riet RP, Vroemen JPAM, Eygendaal D. The epidemiology of radial head fractures. J Shoulder Elb Surg. 2010;19:520–3.
2. Kutscha-Lissberg F, Platzer P, Thalhammer G, Krumböck A, Vécsei V, Braunsteiner T. Incidence and analysis of simultaneous bilateral radial head and neck fractures at a level I trauma center. J Trauma. 2010;69:907–12.
3. Morgan SJ, Groshen SL, Itamura JM, Shankwiler J, Brien WW, Kuschner SH. Reliability evaluation of classifying radial head fractures by the system of Mason. Bull Hosp Jt Dis. 1997;56(2):95–8.
4. Marsh JL, Slongo TF, Agel J, Broderick JS, Creevey W, Decoster TA, Prokuski L, Sirkin MS, Ziran B, Henley B, Audigé L. Fracture and dislocation classification compendium – 2007: Orthopaedic trauma association classification, database and outcomes committee. J Orthop Trauma. 2007;21:S1–6.
5. Johnston GW. A follow-up of one hundred cases of fracture of the head of the radius with a review of the literature. Ulster Med J. 1962;31:51–6. Ulster Medical Society.
6. Iannuzzi NP, Leopold SS. In brief: the Mason classification of radial head fractures. Clin Orthop Relat Res. 2012;470(6):1799–802. Springer-Verlag.
7. van Riet RP, Morrey BF. Documentation of associated injuries occurring with radial head fracture. Clin Orthop Relat Res. 2008;466(1):130–4. Springer-Verlag.
8. Hotchkiss R. Displaced fractures of the radial head: internal fixation or excision? J Am Acad Orthop Surg. 1997;5:1–10.
9. Doornberg J, Elsner A, Kloen P, Marti RK, van Dijk CN, Ring D. Apparently isolated partial articular fractures of the radial head: prevalence and reliability of radiographically diagnosed displacement. J Shoulder Elb Surg. 2007;16:603–8.
10. King GJ, Evans DC, Kellam JF. Open reduction and internal fixation of radial head fractures. J Orthop Trauma. 1991;5:21–8.

11. Holdsworth BJ, Clement DA, Rothwell PN. Fractures of the radial head – the benefit of aspiration: a prospective controlled trial. Injury. 1987;18:44–7.
12. Benson EC, Athwal GS, GJW K. Clinical assessment of the elbow. In: Stanley D, Trail IA, editors. Operative elbow surgery. Edinburgh: Elsevier Churchill Livingstone; 2012. p. 45–66.
13. Norell HG. Roentgenologic visualization of the extracapsular fat; its importance in the diagnosis of traumatic injuries to the elbow. Acta Radiol. 1954;42:205–10.
14. Greenspan A, Norman A. The radial head, capitellum view: useful technique in elbow trauma. AJR Am J Roentgenol. 1982;138(6):1186–8. https://doi.org/10.2214/ajr.138.6.1186.
15. Davidson PA, Moseley JBJ, Tullos HS. A potentially complex injury. Clin Orthop Relat Res. 1993;(297):224–30.
16. Smith AM, Urbanosky LR, Castle JA, Rushing JT, Ruch DS. Radius pull test: predictor of longitudinal forearm instability. J Bone Joint Surg Am. 2002;84(11):1970–6. The American Orthopedic Association.
17. Guitton TG, Brouwer K, Lindenhovius ALC, Dyer G, Zurakowski D, Mudgal CS, Ring DC. Diagnostic accuracy of two-dimensional and three-dimensional imaging and modeling of radial head fractures. J Hand Microsurg. 2013;6:13–7.
18. Laugharne E, Porter KM. Fractures of the radial head and neck. Trauma. 2009;11:249–58.
19. Haverstock JP, Katchky RN, Lalone EA, Faber KJ, King GJW, Athwal GS. Regional variations in radial head bone volume and density: implications for fracture patterns and fixation. J Shoulder Elb Surg. 2012;21:1669–73.
20. van Riet RP, Morrey BF, Driscoll SW, Van Glabbeek F. Associated injuries complicating radial head fractures: a demographic study. Clin Orthop Relat Res. 2005;441:351–5.
21. Kaas L, Turkenburg JL, van Riet RP, Vroemen JPAM, Eygendaal D. Magnetic resonance imaging findings in 46 elbows with a radial head fracture. Acta Orthop. 2010;81(3):373–6. Taylor & Francis.
22. Kaas L, van Riet RP, Vroemen JPAM, Eygendaal D. The incidence of associated fractures of the upper limb in fractures of the radial head. Strategies Trauma Limb Reconstr. 2008;3(2):71–4. Springer Milan.
23. Capo JT, Shamian B, Francisco R, Tan V, Preston JS, Uko L, Yoon RS, Liporace FA. Fracture pattern characteristics and associated injuries of high-energy, large fragment, partial articular radial head fractures: a preliminary imaging analysis. J Orthopaed Traumatol. 2014;16:125–31.
24. King GJW, Zarzour ZDS, Patterson SD, Johnson JA. An anthropometric study of the radial head. J Arthroplast. 2001;16:112–6.
25. Caputo AE, Mazzocca AD, Santoro VM. The nonarticulating portion of the radial head: anatomic and clinical correlations for internal fixation. J Hand Surg Am. 1998;23:1082–90.
26. Smith GR, Hotchkiss RN. Radial head and neck fractures: anatomic guidelines for proper placement of internal fixation. J Shoulder Elb Surg. 1996;5:113–7.
27. Yamaguchi K, Sweet FA, Bindra R, Morrey BF, Gelberman RH. The extraosseous and intraosseous arterial anatomy of the adult elbow. J Bone Joint Surg Am. 1997;79(11):1653–62.
28. Morrey BF, An KN. Articular and ligamentous contributions to the stability of the elbow joint. Am J Sports Med. 1983;11(5):315–9. American Orthopaedic Society for Sports Medicine.
29. Amis AA, Dowson D, Wright V. Elbow joint force predictions for some strenuous isometric actions. J Biomech. 1980;13:765–75.
30. Halls AA, Travill A. Transmission of pressures across the elbow joint. Anat Rec. 1964;150:243–7. Wiley Subscription Services, Inc., A Wiley Company.
31. Morrey BF, An K-N. Stability of the elbow: osseous constraints. J Shoulder Elb Surg. 2005;14:S174–8.
32. Morrey BF, An KN, Stormont TJ. Force transmission through the radial head. J Bone Joint Surg Am. 1988;70(2):250–6. The American Orthopedic Association.
33. Morrey BF, Tanaka S, An K-N. Valgus stability of the elbow: a definition of primary and secondary constraints. Clin Orthop Relat Res. 1991;265:187–95.
34. Johnson JA, Beingessner DM, Gordon KD, Dunning CE, Stacpoole RA, King GJW. Kinematics and stability of the fractured and implant-reconstructed radial head. J Shoulder Elb Surg. 2005;14:S195–201.
35. Jensen SL, Olsen BS, Søjbjerg JO. Elbow joint kinematics after excision of the radial head. J Shoulder Elb Surg. 1999;8:238–41.
36. Beingessner DM, Dunning CE, Beingessner CJ, Johnson JA, King GJW. The effect of radial head fracture size on radiocapitellar joint stability. Clin Biomech. 2003;18:677–81.
37. Radin EL, Riseborough EJ. Fractures of the radial head. A review of eighty-eight cases and analysis of the indications for excision of the radial head and non-operative treatment. J Bone Joint Surg Am. 1966;48(6):1055–64.
38. Miller GK, Drennan DB, Maylahn DJ. Treatment of displaced segmental radial-head fractures. Long-term follow-up. J Bone Joint Surg Am. 1981;63:712–7.
39. Weseley MS, Barenfeld PA, Eisenstein AL. Closed treatment of isolated radial head fractures. J Trauma Acute Care Surg. 1983;23:36–9.
40. Shulman BS, Lee JH, Liporace FA, Egol KA. Minimally displaced radial head/neck fractures (Mason type-I, OTA types 21A2.2 and 21B2.1): are we "over treating" our patients? J Orthop Trauma. 2015;29:e31–5.
41. Dowdy PA, Bain GI, King GJ, Patterson SD. The midline posterior elbow incision. An anatomical appraisal. J Bone Joint Surg Br. 1995;77(5):696–9.
42. Witt JD, Kamineni S. The posterior interosseous nerve and the posterolateral approach to the proximal radius. J Bone Joint Surg Br. 1998;80(2):240–2.

43. Kocher T. Text-book of operative surgery. New York: Macmillan; 1913.
44. Kaplan EB. Surgical approach to the proximal end of the radius and its use in fractures of the head and neck of the radius. J Bone Joint Surg. 1941;23:86–92.
45. Cheung EV, Steinmann SP. Surgical approaches to the elbow. J Am Acad Orthop Surg. 2009;17:325–33. American Academy of Orthopaedic Surgeons.
46. Desloges W, Louati H, Papp SR, Pollock JW. Objective analysis of lateral elbow exposure with the extensor digitorum communis split compared with the kocher interval. J Bone Joint Surg. 2014;96:387–93.
47. Parasa RB, Maffulli N. Surgical management of radial head fractures. J R Coll Surg Edinb. 2001;46:76–85.
48. Goldberg I, Peylan J, Yosipovitch Z. Late results of excision of the radial head for an isolated closed fracture. J Bone Joint Surg Am. 1986;68(5):675–9. The American Orthopedic Association.
49. Yalcinkaya M, Bagatur AE, Erdogan S, Zorer G. Resection arthroplasty for Mason type III radial head fractures yield good clinical but poor radiological results in the long term. Orthopedics. 2013;36(11):e1358–64. SLACK Incorporated.
50. Coleman DA, Blair WF, Shurr D. Resection of the radial head for fracture of the radial head. Long-term follow-up of seventeen cases. J Bone Joint Surg Am. 1987;69(3):385–92.
51. Poehling GG, Whipple TL, Sisco L, Goldman B III. Elbow arthroscopy: a new technique. Arthroscopy. 2010;26:1246–7.
52. Wijeratna M, Bailey KA, Pace A, Tytherleigh-Strong G, Van Rensburg L, Kent M. Arthroscopic radial head excision in managing elbow trauma. International Orthopaedics (SICOT). 2012;36:2507–12.
53. Ring D, Quintero J, Jupiter JB. Open reduction and internal fixation of fractures of the radial head. J Bone Joint Surg Am. 2002;84:1811–5. The American Orthopedic Association.
54. Sanders RA, French HG. Open reduction and internal fixation of comminuted radial head fractures. Am J Sports Med. 1986;14:130–5. Am Orthopaedic Society for Sports Medicine.
55. Zwingmann J, Welzel M, Dovi-Akue D, Schmal H, Südkamp NP, Strohm PC. Clinical results after different operative treatment methods of radial head and neck fractures: a systematic review and meta-analysis of clinical outcome. Injury. 2013;44(11):1540–50.
56. Rolla PR, Surace MF, Bini A, Pilato G. Arthroscopic treatment of fractures of the radial head. Arthroscopy. 2006;22:233.e1–6.
57. Brooks-Hill AL, Regan WD. Extra-articular arthroscopic lateral elbow release. Arthroscopy. 2008;24:483–5.
58. Patterson JD, Jones CK, Glisson RR, Caputo AE, Goetz TJ, Goldner RD. Stiffness of simulated radial neck fractures fixed with 4 different devices. J Shoulder Elb Surg. 2001;10:57–61.
59. Robert Giffin J, King GJW, Patterson SD, Johnson JA. Internal fixation of radial neck fractures: an in vitro biomechanical analysis. Clin Biomech. 2004;19:358–61.
60. Smith AM, Morrey BF, Steinmann SP. Low profile fixation of radial head and neck fractures: surgical technique and clinical experience. J Orthop Trauma. 2007;21:718–24.
61. Itamura J, Roidis N, Mirzayan R, Vaishnav S, Learch T, Shean C. Radial head fractures: MRI evaluation of associated injuries. J Shoulder Elb Surg. 2005;14:421–4.
62. Caputo AE, Burton KJ, Cohen MS, King GJ. Articular cartilage injuries of the capitellum interposed in radial head fractures: a report of ten cases. J Shoulder Elb Surg. 2006;15:716–20.
63. King GJ, Zarzour ZD, Rath DA, Dunning CE, Patterson SD, Johnson JA. Metallic radial head arthroplasty improves valgus stability of the elbow. Clin Orthop Relat Res. 1999;368:114–25.
64. Shannon HL, Deluce SR, Giles JW, Johnson JA, King GJW. The effect of radial head implant shape on radiocapitellar kinematics during in vitro forearm rotation. J Shoulder Elbow Surg. 2015;24(2):258–64. Elsevier.
65. Harrington IJ, Sekyi-Otu A, Barrington TW, Evans DC, Tuli V. The functional outcome with metallic radial head implants in the treatment of unstable elbow fractures: a long-term review. J Trauma. 2001;50:46–52.
66. Popovic N, Lemaire R, Georis P, Gillet P. Midterm results with a bipolar radial head prosthesis: radiographic evidence of loosening at the bone-cement interface. J Bone Joint Surg Am. 2007;89(11):2469–76. The Journal of Bone and Joint Surgery, Inc.
67. Chanlalit C, Shukla DR, Fitzsimmons JS, Thoreson AR, An K-N, Driscoll SW. Radiocapitellar stability: the effect of soft tissue integrity on bipolar versus monopolar radial head prostheses. J Shoulder Elb Surg. 2011;20:219–25.
68. Abdulla I, Langohr GDG, Gladwell M, Yeung C, Faber KJ, King GJW, Athwal GS. The effect of fracture comminution on the reliability and accuracy of radial head sizing. J Shoulder Elbow Surg, vol. 2015;24(3):364–8. Elsevier.
69. Doornberg JN, Linzel DS, Zurakowski D, Ring D. Reference points for radial head prosthesis size. J Hand Surg Am. 2006;31(1):53–7.
70. Frank SG, Grewal R, Johnson J, Faber KJ, King GJ, Athwal GS. Determination of correct implant size in radial head arthroplasty to avoid overlengthening. J Bone Joint Surg Am. 2000;91(7):1738–46.
71. Birkedal JP, Deal DN, Ruch DS. Loss of flexion after radial head replacement. J Shoulder Elb Surg. 2004;13:208–13.
72. Grewal R, MacDermid JC, Faber KJ, Drosdowech DS, King GJW. Comminuted radial head fractures treated with a modular metallic radial head arthroplasty. J Bone Joint Surg Am. 2006;88(10):2192–200. The Journal of Bone and Joint Surgery, Inc.
73. Thompson HC, Garcia A. Myositis ossificans: aftermath of elbow injuries. Clin Orthop Relat Res. 1967;50:129–34.

74. Coonrad RW, Roush TF, Major NM, Basamania CJ. The drop sign, a radiographic warning sign of elbow instability. J Shoulder Elb Surg. 2005;14:312–7.
75. Lee AT, Schrumpf MA, Choi D, Meyers KN, Patel R, Wright TM, Hotchkiss RN, Daluiski A. The influence of gravity on the unstable elbow. J Shoulder Elb Surg. 2013;22:81–7.
76. Mason ML. Some observations on fractures of the head of the radius with a review of one hundred cases. Br J Surg. 1954;42(172):123–32. John Wiley & Sons, Ltd.
77. Akesson T, Herbertsson P, Josefsson PO, Hasserius R, Besjakov J, Karlsson MK. Primary nonoperative treatment of moderately displaced two-part fractures of the radial head. J Bone Joint Surg Am. 2006;88(9):1909–14. The Journal of Bone and Joint Surgery, Inc.
78. Duckworth AD, Wickramasinghe NR, Clement ND, Court-Brown CM, McQueen MM. Long-term outcomes of isolated stable radial head fractures. J Bone Joint Surg Am. 2014;96(20):1716–23. The American Orthopedic Association.
79. Smits AJ, Giannakopoulos GF, Zuidema WP. Long-term results and treatment modalities of conservatively treated Broberg-Morrey type 1 radial head fractures. Injury. 2014;45:1564–8. Elsevier.
80. Duckworth AD, Clement ND, Jenkins PJ, Will EM, Court-Brown CM, McQueen MM. Socioeconomic deprivation predicts outcome following radial head and neck fractures. Injury. 2012;43:1102–6.
81. Broberg MA, Morrey BF. Results of delayed excision of the radial head after fracture. J Bone Joint Surg Am. 1986;68:669–74.
82. Miki AD, Vukadinovi SM. Late results in fractures of the radial head treated by excision. Clin Orthop Relat Res. 1983;181:220–8.
83. Edwards GSJ, Jupiter JB. Radial head fractures with acute distal radioulnar dislocation: Essex-Lopresti revisited. Clin Orthop Relat Res. 1988;234:61–9.
84. Trousdale RT, Amadio PC, Cooney WP, Morrey BF. Radio-ulnar dissociation. A review of twenty cases. J Bone Joint Surg Am. 1992;74:1486–97.
85. Ikeda M, Sugiyama K, Kang C, Takagaki T, Oka Y. Comminuted fractures of the radial head. J Bone Joint Surg Am. 2005;87:76–84. The American Orthopedic Association.
86. Menth-Chiari WA, Ruch DS, Poehling GG. Arthroscopic excision of the radial head: clinical outcome in 12 patients with post-traumatic arthritis after fracture of the radial head or rheumatoid arthritis. Arthroscopy. 2001;17(9):918–23.
87. Hall JA, McKee MD. Posterolateral rotatory instability of the elbow following radial head resection. J Bone Joint Surg Am. 2005;87(7):1571–9. The American Orthopedic Association.
88. Garland DE, Hanscom DA, Keenan MA, Smith C, Moore T. Resection of heterotopic ossification in the adult with head trauma. J Bone Joint Surg Am. 1985;67:1261–9.
89. Gaston SR, Smith FM, Baab OD. Adult injuries of the radial head and neck; importance of time element in treatment. Am J Surg. 1949;78(5):631–5.
90. Lindenhovius ALC, Felsch Q, Doornberg JN, Ring D, Kloen P. Open reduction and internal fixation compared with excision for unstable displaced fractures of the radial head. J Hand Surg Am. 2007;32(5):630–6.
91. Zarattini G, Galli S, Marchese M, Mascio LD, Pazzaglia UE. The surgical treatment of isolated Mason type 2 fractures of the radial head in adults: comparison between radial head resection and open reduction and internal fixation. J Orthop Trauma. 2012;26:229–35.
92. Yoon A, King GJW, Grewal R. Is ORIF superior to nonoperative treatment in isolated displaced partial articular fractures of the radial head? Clin Orthop Relat Res. 2014;472:2105–12.
93. Pike JM, Grewal R, Athwal GS, Faber KJ, King GJW. Open reduction and internal fixation of radial head fractures: do outcomes differ between simple and complex injuries? Clin Orthop Relat Res. 2014;472:2120–7.
94. Watters TS, Garrigues GE, Ring D, Ruch DS. Fixation versus replacement of radial head in terrible triad: is there a difference in elbow stability and prognosis? Clin Orthop Relat Res. 2014;472:2128–35.
95. Leigh WB, Ball CM. Radial head reconstruction versus replacement in the treatment of terrible triad injuries of the elbow. J Shoulder Elb Surg. 2012;21:1336–41.
96. Shukla DR, Pillai G, McAnany S, Hausman M, Parsons BO. Heterotopic ossification formation after fracture-dislocations of the elbow. J Shoulder Elb Surg. 2015;24:333–8.
97. Moro JK, Werier J, MacDermid JC, Patterson SD, King GJ. Arthroplasty with a metal radial head for unreconstructible fractures of the radial head. J Bone Joint Surg (Am Vol). 2001;83-A(8):1201–11.
98. Ruan H-J, Fan C-Y, Liu J-J, B-F Z. A comparative study of internal fixation and prosthesis replacement for radial head fractures of Mason type III. Int Orthop. 2009;33(1):249–53. Springer-Verlag.
99. Chen X, S-C W, Cao L-h, G-Q Y, Li M, J-C S. Comparison between radial head replacement and open reduction and internal fixation in clinical treatment of unstable, multi-fragmented radial head fractures. Int Orthop. 2011;35(7):1071–6. Springer-Verlag.
100. Van Glabbeek F, Van Riet RP, Baumfeld JA, Neale PG, O'Driscoll SW, Morrey BF, An KN. Detrimental effects of overstuffing or Understuffing with a radial head replacement in the medial collateral-ligament deficient elbow. J Bone Joint Surg Am. 2004;86(12):2629–35. The American Orthopedic Association.

101. Duckworth AD, Wickramasinghe NR, Clement ND, Court-Brown CM, McQueen MM. Radial head replacement for acute complex fractures: what are the rate and risks factors for revision or removal? Clin Orthop Relat Res. 2014;472:2136–43.
102. Flinkkilä T, Kaisto T, Sirniö K, Hyvönen P, Leppilahti J. Short- to mid-term results of metallic press-fit radial head arthroplasty in unstable injuries of the elbow. J Bone Joint Surg Br. 2012;94(6):805–10.
103. Stuffmann E, Gannon A, Clemente J, Baratz M. Radial head prosthesis update. Tech Shoulder Elb Surg. 2009;10(1):31–8.
104. Herald J, Driscoll S. Complete dissociation of a bipolar radial head prosthesis: a case report. J Shoulder Elb Surg. 2008;17:e22–3.

Monteggia Fractures and Monteggia-Like-Lesions

6

Karl Braun, Gunter H. Sandmann, Martin Lucke, and Moritz Crönlein

Abbreviations

RH	Radial head
MCL	Medial collateral ligament
ROM	Range of motion
ORIF	Open reduction and internal fixation

Epidemiology and Background

While the elbow is the second most commonly dislocated joint in adults, Monteggia fractures and Monteggia-like-lesions remain rare and complex entities, approximately accounting for 2–7% of all proximal forearm fractures and 0.7% of all elbow fractures and dislocations [1–4]. Monteggia fractures are defined as an ulnar-based forearm fracture in combination with a proximal radioulnar joint/radial head dislocation and are always designated as complex. This injury pattern has first been described by Giovanni Battista Monteggia in 1814 and was further characterized by Luis Bado in 1967 [5, 6]. Bado introduced a classification system of four subtypes according to the mechanism of injury and the corresspondent fracture pattern of the ulna [3]. Of these four subtypes, Jesse Jupiter, further classified the posterior Monteggia lesion (Bado type II) in 1991 depending on the location and type of ulnar fracture as well as the pattern of radial head injury [7, 8]. In addition to these original Monteggia fractures, several Monteggia-like lesions/equivalents have been described based on the similarity of their proposed injury mechanism [3].

Importand requirements for the achievement of good results following the Monteggia fracture or Monteggia-like lesion are: firstly, an early detection of the fracture type; secondly, an open reduction and internal stable fixation of the ulna; thirdly, a mostly open reduction of the radial head; and finally, short immobilization time [9]. Nevertheless, despite a better understanding of the biomechanical principles and advances in surgical treatment options, Monteggia and Monteggia-like lesions are still frequently associated with complications, poor functional outcomes, and high rates of revision surgery [1, 10].

K. Braun (✉)
Department of Trauma Surgery, University Hospital Rechts der Isar, Technical University Munich, Munich, Germany
e-mail: karl.braun@mri.tum.de

G. H. Sandmann
Department of Trauma Surgery, University Hospital Rechts der Isar, Technical University Munich, Munich, Germany

Sportklinik Ravensburg, Ravensburg, Germany

M. Lucke
Surgical Clinic Munich South, Munich, Germany

M. Crönlein
Department of Trauma Surgery, Klinikum rechts der Isar, Munich, Germany

P. Biberthaler et al. (eds.), *Acute Elbow Trauma*, Strategies in Fracture Treatments,
https://doi.org/10.1007/978-3-319-97850-5_6

Classification

Monteggia

The original Monteggia fracture was described as a *proximal-third ulna fracture with an associated radial head dislocation*. However, this simple description has been further elaborated and evalutated through various classification schemes [11]. However, none of these classification schemes are exhaustive, and most of them have little therapeutic or prognostic value. Monteggia-like, Monteggia-equivalent, and Monteggia-variant lesions and trans-olecranon fracture-dislocations get frequently confused, and it can prove very difficult to classify some lesions correctly using current classifications [12–14].

Bado Classification

The Bado classification remains the best known classification of Monteggia fracures, linking the mechanism of injury to the direction of radial head displacement. The classification depends on the direction of the radial head's dislocation and the angulation of the fracture of the ulna [3]. **Type I** describes a dislocation of the radial head in anterior direction and the typical trauma mechanism is forced pronation of the forearm along with hyperextension of the elbow. A type II injury consists of a proximal or middle-third ulna fracture with a posteior or postero-lateral dislocation of the radial head and is usually caused by axial loading on a partially flexed elbow. A fall on the elbow with hyperextension and pronation in combination with forced abduction or varus stress results in a type III injury. This injury consists of a fracture of the metaphyseal ulna with lateral or anterolateral dislocation of the radial head. A Bado type IV fracture is a proximal- or middle-third ulna fracture along with anterior dislocation of the radial head and fracture of the proximal third of the radius. The trauma mechanism of this injury is comparable to that of type I fractures, however, a result of higher energy/greater impact (Fig. 6.1) [11]. Type II injuries are most common accounting for about 80% of all Monteggia fractures, followed by type I (15%) and type III and IV (5% combined) [15, 16].

Jupiter Classification

While Bado primarily focuses on the radial component, Jupiter modified his classification as follows: in order to guide necessary treatment strategies, Jesse Jupiter defined subtypes for the posterior Monteggia fractures (Bado type II) into four subtypes on the basis of the location and type of ulna fracture sustained as well as the pattern of radial head injury [7, 17]. **Type IIA** fractures involve the most proximal aspect of the ulna (olecranon) and the coronoid process. **Type IIB** fractures occur at the ulnar metaphyseal-diaphyseal junction, distal to the coronoid process. **Type IIC** fracture occur at the diaphyseal level and **type IID** fractures are comminuted extending from the olecranon to the ulnar diaphysis (Fig. 6.2).

Monteggia-Like Lesions

The eponym of Monteggia fracture includes various patterns of complex fracture-dislocations of the proximal ulna and radius which are not well defined yet [8]. In Monteggia-like lesions radial head fractures are classified according to Mason's modified classifications [18–20]. Each radial head fracture type must be adequately recognized and addressed. The varying combinations of these injured structures explains the complexity and diversity of the management procedures (Fig. 6.3).

Proximal Ulnar and Radial Fracture-Dislocation Comprehensive Classification System (PURCCS)

One of the latest classification schemes incorporating current research and knowledge about the functional anatomy of the elbow is the PURCCS scheme [12]. This scheme includes the complex interaction between bone and soft-tissue constraints of the joint and aims to guide therapeutic decisions. However, even with this detailed classification the various subgroubs cannot always be sharply differentiated.

The classification is based on specific anatomic injuries, defined as the "main lesions", including (1) level of ulnar fracture (with respect to collateral

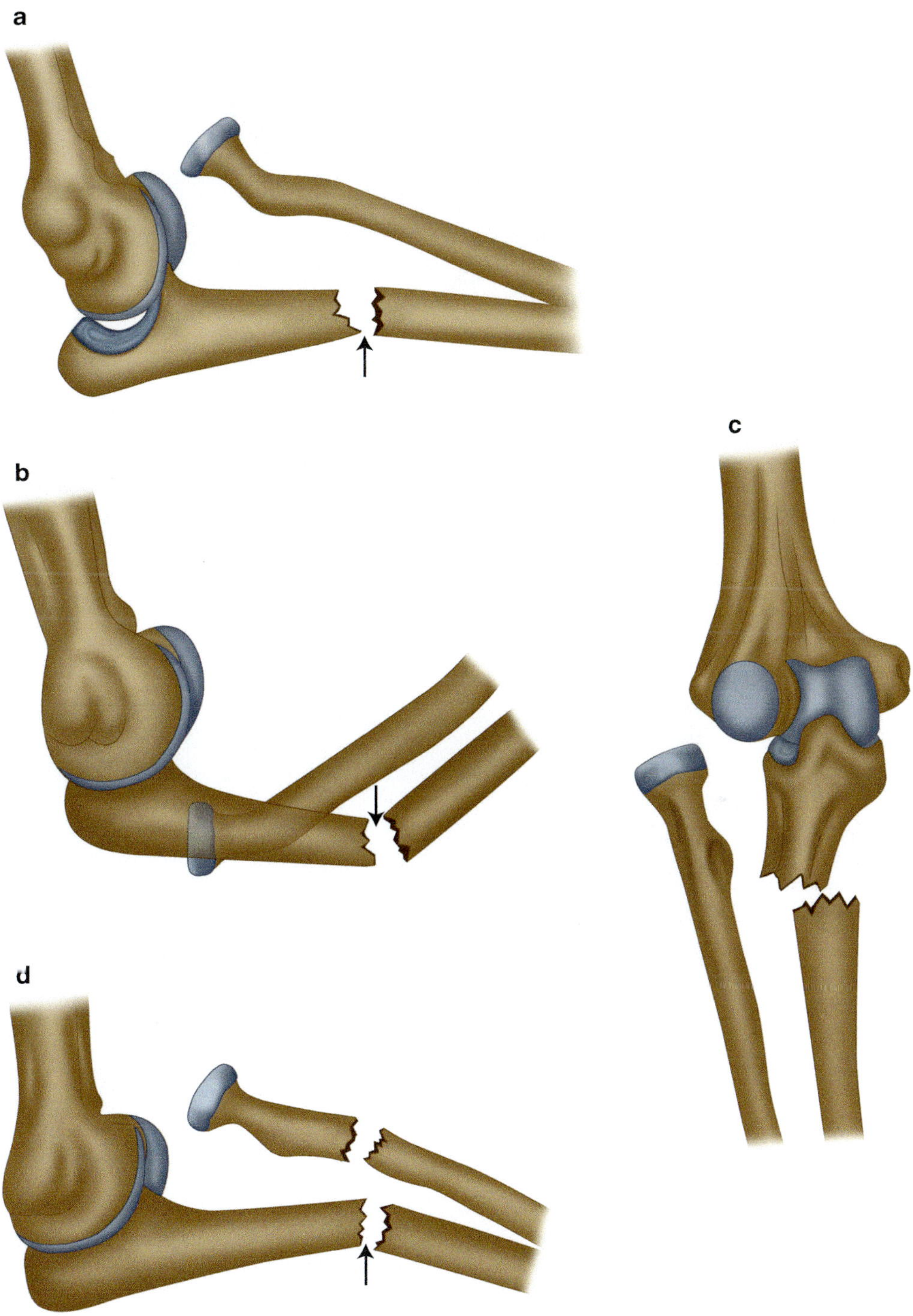

Fig. 6.1 Bado classification of Monteggia fractures: (**a**) Bado Type I anterior dislocation of the radial head, (**b**) Bado Type II posterior/posterolateral dislocation of the radial head, (**c**) Bado Type III lateral dislocation of the radial head, and (**d**) Bado Type IV anterior dislocation of the radial head along with fracture of the proximal radius [11]

ligament insertion and coronoid process), (2) radiohumeral dislocation, (3) proximal radioulnar dislocation, (4) radial fracture, (5) distal radioulnar and interosseous membrane lesion, and (6) ulnohumeral dislocation. Furthermore, ulnar fracture was labeled with numbers [1–6], and the presence of

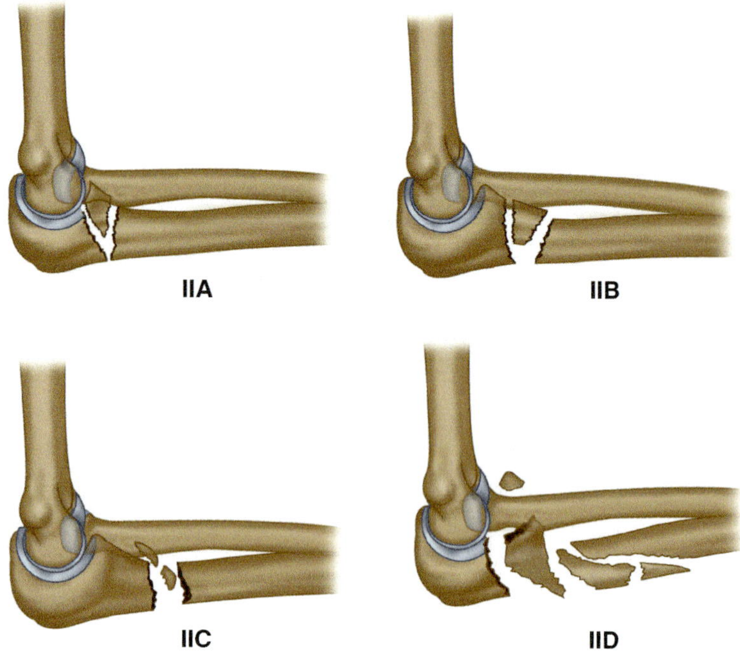

Fig. 6.2 Radial head fracture, which are common in Bado type II fractures as the radial head shears against the capitellum during posterior dislocation, are classified in four types: 0 = no fracture; 1 = one part fracture; 2 = two part fracture; 3 = comminuted [11]

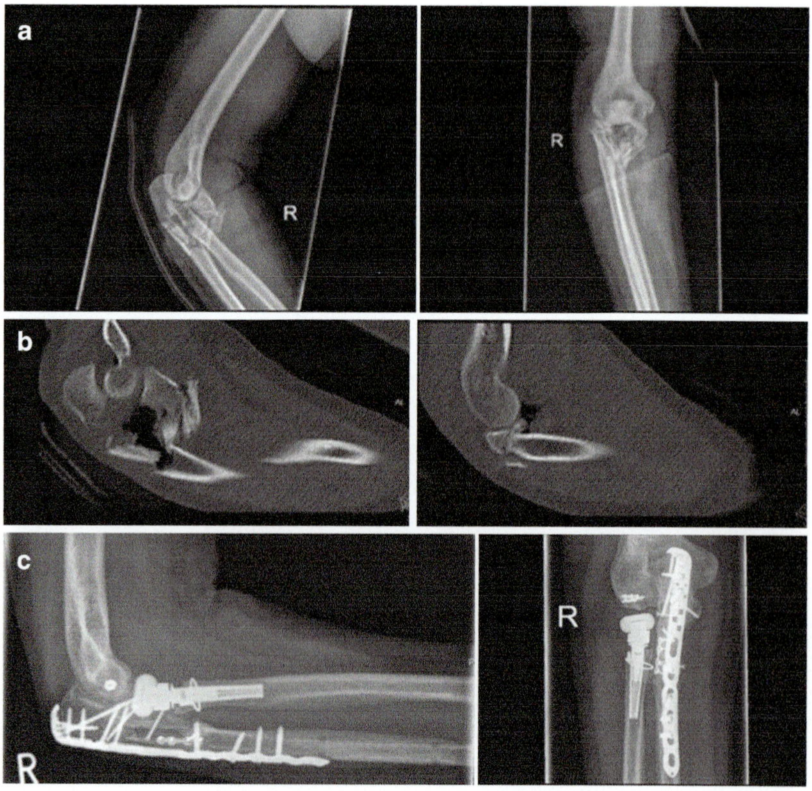

Fig. 6.3 Example of a Monteggia-like lesion; Jupiter IID. (**a**) x-ray a.p. and lateral view; (**b**) CT scan revealing the comminuted fracture with destruction of the coronoid and dislocation of the radial head; (**c**) postoperative result after radial head replacement (MoPyC, Fa. Tornier), radial stabilization and ulnar plating

elbow joint dislocation, distal radioulnar dislocation and radial fracture was labeled with letters (A-E). The direction of dislocation and the type of radial fracture were labeled with Roman numerals (I-III) placed after the letter. The progression of the alphabetic and numeric codes indicates an increase in complexity of the lesion and, thus, in the treatment (Fig. 6.4) [12, 21].

Symptoms and Diagnostics

A fall onto the extended outstretched hand with an overwhelming axial force is usually described as the mechanism of injury [22]. Patients will most often present immediately after trauma with pain, edema and swelling, tenderness, decreased range and/or restriction of motion, and commonly deformity about the forearm [2, 23].

An initial neurovascular examination is the first "must-do" before any further manipulation/treatment of the elbow. In order to accurately evaluate the injury pattern and thus plan the necessary therapeutic steps, a thorough and most of all, standardized diagnostic approach should be conducted. Neurovascular examination is always the first „must-do "before any further manipulation/treatment of the elbow. Anteroposterior and lateral standard radiographs as well as a computerized tomography scans (with 3D reconstruction) are needed to properly evaluate the severity of bone injuries [11, 24].

Injury Pattern and Surgery Related Anatomy

A precise understanding of the anatomic contributors to the elbow stability as well as the biomechanics of the fracture pattern is essential to treat these complex lesions [9, 25]. One of the primary treatment goals of monteggia fractures are the restoration of the normal contour and dimension of the ulnar length, coronoid process height, and trochlear notch to restore stability [26, 27]. The unique bony architecture of the proximal ulna shaft with its anteromedial varus angulation in the proximal third, needs to be strictly reduced due to its great importance for the maintenance of the articular geometry of the elbow with special respect of the proximal articulation of the radius [22, 28].

Regarding the mechanism of injury, direct force from the dorsal side is the usual mechanism of injury for **Bado type I** fractures: a fracture of the ulna occurs due to a direct force of the proximal ulna; the radial head dislocates to its ventral side [29]. An axial force to the 90° bent elbow leads to a **Bado type II** fracture as a variation of the posterior elbow dislocation [30]. A simultaneous pronation of the forearm in combination with an abduction force leads to a **Bado type III** fracture most frequently with a ventrolateral dislocation of the radial head [31]. The exact mechanism of injury for **Bado type IV** fractures is unknown [2].

In order to properly treat Monteggia lesions, a posterior approach with the patient in a prone position is recommended. In most cases, the radial head realigns after the anatomical reconstruction of the ulna with no further need for an open reduction of the radial head. If the dislocation of the radial head persists after ulnar reduction, the surgeon must re-evaluate the ulnar alignment with special respect to ulnar length and vaus angulation [32].

For Monteggia-like lesions also, a single posterior approach is favourable. The radial head fracture can be addressed from behind "through" the ulnar fracture after mobilization of the anconeus muscle. The operative algorithm should then address any fracture of the coronoid process followed by the ulnar shaft. For better visualizatio of the coronoid it might be necessary to use an additional medial approach or a ventral approach in order to anatomically reduce the fracture [33]. Possible ligament reconstructions should be performed last [2, 33, 34].

Therapeutic Options

Monteggia lesions can be treated in an operative or conservative manner, depending on fracture type, age of the patients and time of reduction [35]. Figure 6.5 provides a possible treatment

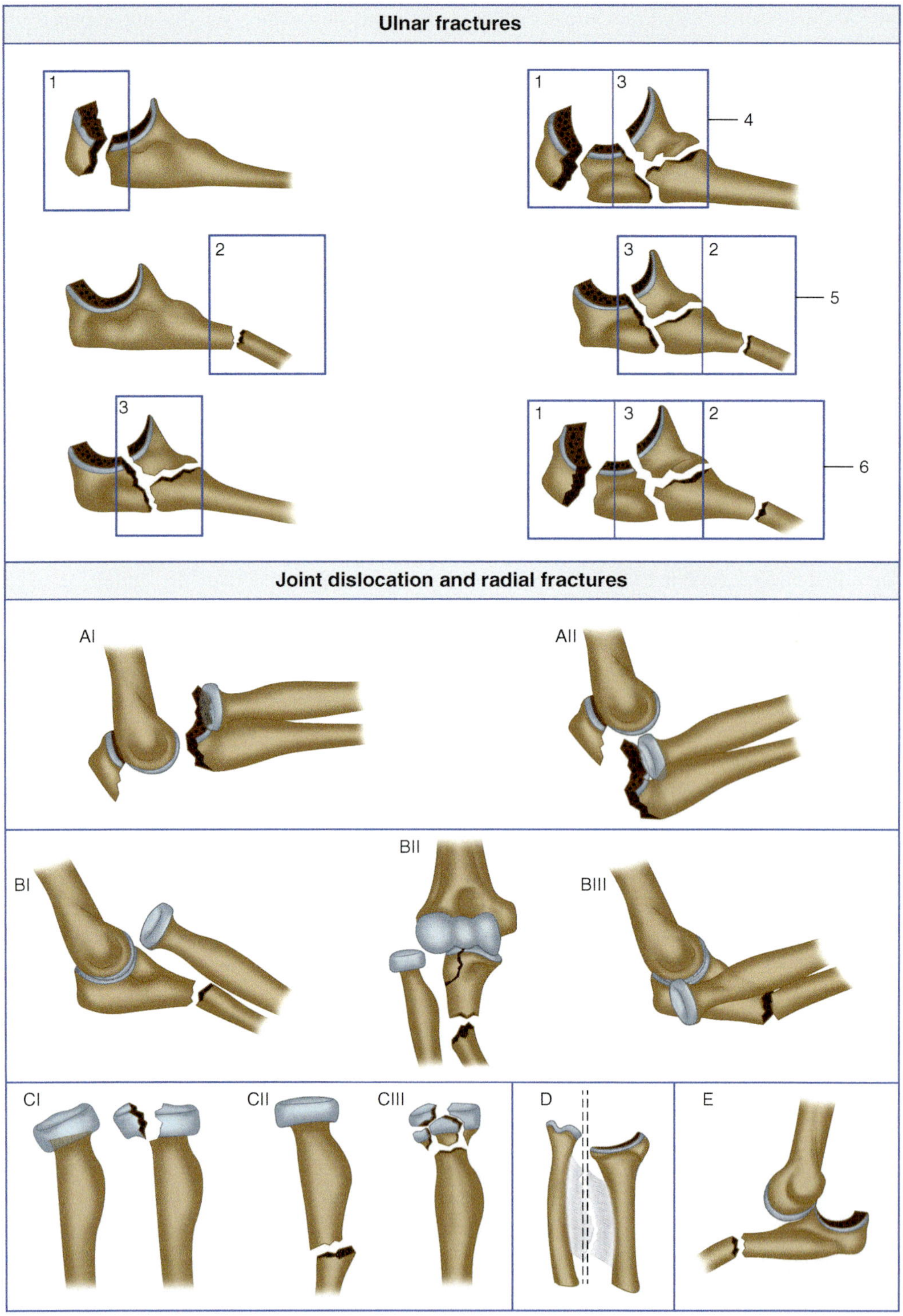

Fig. 6.4 PURCCS scheme. Ulnar fracture type was labeled with numbers [1–6], and the presence of elbow joint dislocations, distal radioulnar dislocation, and or radial fracture was labeled with letters (A-E). The direction of dislocation and the type of radial fracture were labeled with Roman numerals (I-III) placed after the letter [17]

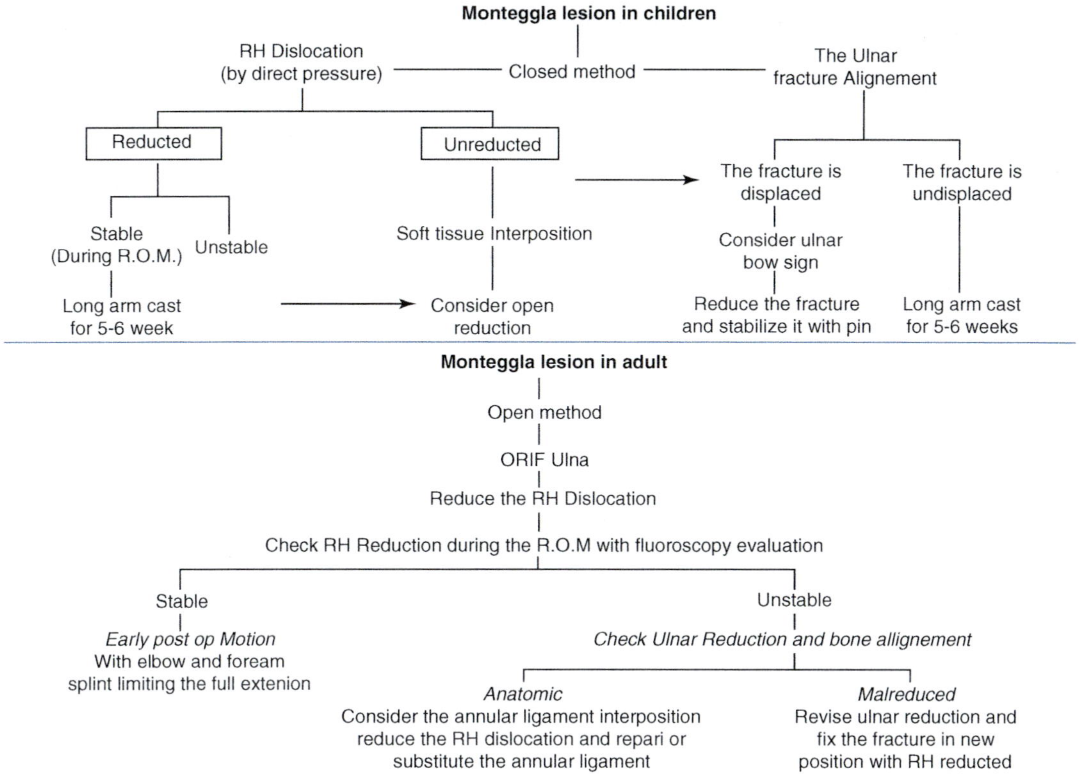

Fig. 6.5 Age dependent treatment algorithm for Monteggia lesions [35]

Table 6.1 Treatment algorithm for acute Monteggia fracture dislocations based on ulnar fracture pattern [36]

Ulnar fracture pattern	Treatment
Plastic deformation	Closed reduction, casting
Greenstick (incomplete) fracture	Closed reduction, casting
Transverse or short oblique complete fracture	Closed reduction, intramedullary fixation
Long oblique or comminuted fracture	Open reduction and plate fixation

algorithm for Monteggia fractures based on the patients' age to simplify decision making in treating these complex elbow injuries (see Fig. 6.5).

Nonoperative Treatment

In general, nonoperative treatment of Monteggia fractures and Monteggia-like lesions with closed reduction followed by splint stabilization is only recommended in very few cases in children [35, 36]. In adults, closed reduction is only to be considered in the emergency room for initial assessment. Definite operative treatment should be obtained as soon as possible. Principles of conservative treatment are similar to the operative strategies. The ulnar alignment and length has to be restored first, followed by closed reduction of the radial head (RH) displacement [37]. Due to the importance of the correct ulnar length and alignment, conservative treatment can only be recommended in stable ulna fractures that can maintain their alignment after reduction. This only counts for plastic deformations or Greenstick fractures. In transverse or short oblique fractures of the ulna, the correct ulnar length and alignment might be achieved by minimally invasive intramedullary pinning instead. A treatment algorithm based on the ulnar fracture pattern in children had been published by Ring and Waters (see Table 6.1) [36, 38].

For closed reduction in children usually general anaesthesia is necessary to avoid any pain during the reposition. The reposition manoeuvre should be performed under fluoroscopy to verify congruent radiohumeral joint reduction and correct ulnar alignment [39]. After restoring correct ulnar length via longitudinal traction, direct pressure on the radial head during elbow flexion over 90° and supination is used to restore the correct joint alignment. To maintain the correct alignment, the elbow should be stabilized in a cast in 110–120° flexion and supination [39]. Definite anteroposterior and lateral X-rays following reposition are necessary to control the correct joint congruency [35]. A bivalve cast therapy in midrotation to reduce traction of the biceps tendon should be obtained for 4–5 weeks [35, 39]. Serial radiographs and neurovascular check-ups are recommended at least 4, 7 and 11 days after reposition to ascertain maintenance of the correct alignment [39]. Gentle range of motion exercises to avoid stiffness of the elbow joint can be performed after clinically and radiologically confirmed fracture healing [39].

Operative Treatment

Besides these very few indications for conservative treatment, most of the Monteggia fractures and Monteggia-like lesions need to be treated in an operative manner. The main treatment principles are [16]:

1. Open reduction and anatomical restoration of the ulna fracture, followed by reposition of the RH (Fig. 6.6)
2. Treatment of concomitant injuries (RH fractures, coronoid fractures, LCL ruptures etc.)

For operative treatment, the patient is placed in lateral decubital or supine position with an tourniquet placed on the upper arm [35, 9]. A posterior mid-line or posterolateral approach is recommended because it gives a good overview and can be used to expose both, the ulna/olecranon and the RH at the same time. Gold standard for reduction of the ulnar fracture in adults is plate and screw fixation [39], however tension-band wiring can still be considered in simple oblique fractures especially when they are located proximally [9, 40]. To restore ulnar length in children, intramedullary pinning can be performed, if the ulnar fracture allows biomechanically stable pinning [41].

After restoring correct ulnar length and rotation, the RH can usually be reduced easily. The annular ligament should be treated by suture to give additional stability [9]. An intraoperative stability check should be performed under fluoroscopy.

In Monteggia-like lesions, concomitant injuries can aggravate the operative treatment. In cases of additional displaced RH fractures (Mason type II-IV), the RH should be reduced by screw or plate fixation using the Kocher's interval between the anconeus and extensor carpi ulnaris muscle [42]. In comminuted RH fractures arthroplasty represents an alternative surgical approach with good short to mid-term results and should be preferred prior radial head resection [43].

Additional coronoid fractures enlarge the risk of humero-ulnar translation instability [9]. While stable Regan/Morrey type I coronoid fractures do not require special treatment, type II and III fractures should be addressed by screw fixation, since they cause a high risk of joint instability due to medial collateral ligament (MCL) involvement [9]. Posteriorly- anteriorly placed screws can be used to address the coronoid fracture if the fragments are large enough. If the fragments are too small for screw fixation, suture anchors can be used passed around the coronoid tip including the anterior capsule [39]. The complexity of Monteggia fractures can be seen in Fig. 6.6. A 26-year-old- male patient was referred to our clinic following operative treatment (ORIF and LCP osteosynthesis) of an anterior Monteggia fracture (Bado type 1). The postoperative X-rays and CT scans showed a consisting anterior radial head dislocation. As the fracture of the ulna shaft was obviously malreduced revision surgery was initiated. Even after meticulous reduction of the fracture and plate revision, the radial head subluxation persisted. The patient therefore underwent additional diagnostics (CT Scan/MRI Scan). The 3D-CT-reconstruction of both forearms revealed the problem of the operative treatment and the reason for the persisting radial head subluxation (right: injured arm, left: contralateral arm). Even though,

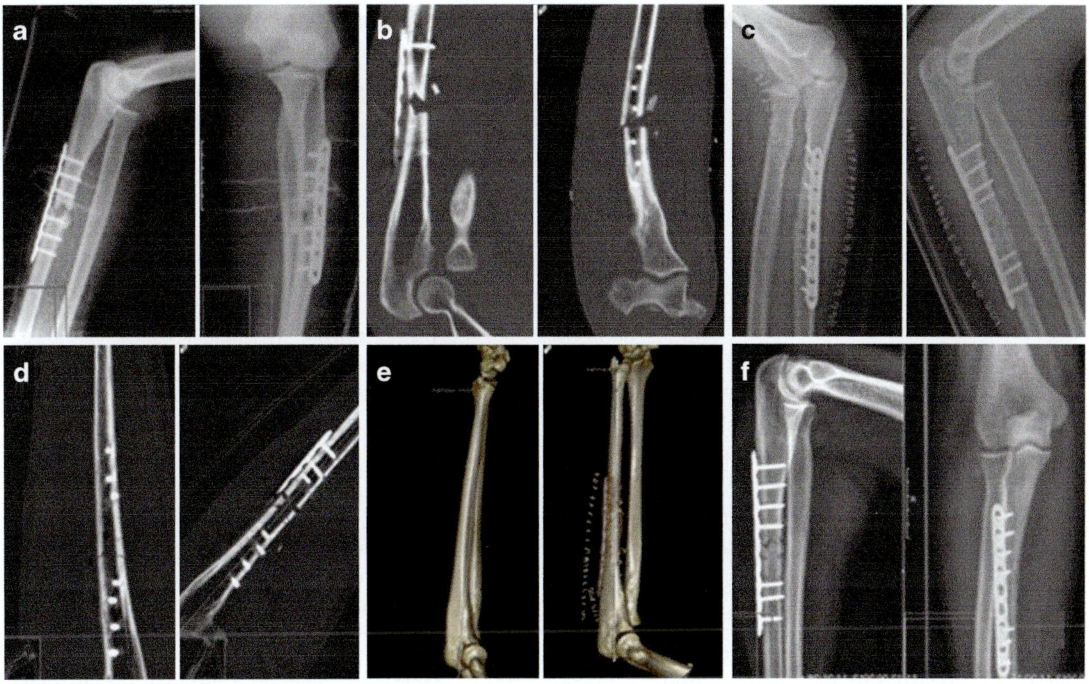

Fig. 6.6 Importance of restoration of the exact ulnar length and rotation. (**a**, **b**) Anterior radial head dislocation following ORIF and LCP osteosynthesis. (**c**) Persisting radial head subluxation following revision surgery with meticulous reduction. (**d**, **e**) Additional diagnostics (CT Scan and 3D-CT reconstruction of both forearms) revealed not assembled ulnar bowing. (**f**) After second revision with restoration of ulnar bowing a well centered humeruo-radial joint could be achieved

fracture reduction appeared anatomically, the ulnar bowing was not assembled analogue to the contralateral arm. Besides prior reconstruction of ulnar length and rotation in a second revision surgery the bowing of the ulna was now corrected. By this correction a well centered humero-radial joint could be achieved with a free range of motion for pro- and supination. This case demonstrates the importance of the anatomical restoration of the ulnar fracture and geometry as a key treatment principle for Monteggia fractures.

Postoperative Care

In paediatric patients, who tolerate immobilization better than adults, the elbow is placed in a bivalved cast in 90° flexion with forearm supination postoperatively. Cast immobilization is recommended for 4–6 weeks. Intramedullary placed K-wires are usually removed 4 weeks after surgery [37, 39].

In contrast to paediatric patients, adults have a high risk of developing postoperative stiffness of the elbow, leading to the fact that the elbow splint should be removed 2–3 days after surgery. Early motion should be initiated, beginning with gravity assisted flexion and extension under physiotherapeutic control 2–3 times a week for at least 6 weeks [9, 35, 39]. The healing process should be evaluated via X-rays 6 weeks postoperatively. If healing could be obtained, physiotherapeutic training with higher loads should be initiated. Maximum loads and return to sports should be avoided for at least 3 months after surgery.

Outcomes and Complications

Functional results following Monteggia fractures and Monteggia-like lesions treated with open reduction and internal fixation (ORIF) vary and show acceptable results in at least 70–83%, depending on the fracture type [44]. Unfortunately, there are numerous complications leading to potential bad outcomes following operative treatment.

Non-union rates account for up to 22% in current literature following ORIF of Monteggia fractures. Persisting pain, leading to early implant removal is described in up to 46% of the patients [44].

Stiffness following ORIF of Monteggia fractures and Monteggia-like lesions is still one of the major complications. While children, even after 4 weeks of immobilization, usually regain their full elbow ROM, adults frequently present with a limited elbow function postoperatively. Therefore, a postoperative protocol with decreased immobilization is highly recommended [37, 39].

Heterotopic ossifications leading to painful ROM restrictions are frequently seen in patients with elbow injuries. While rates of 6–8% are described in patients with simple ulna fractures, heterotopic ossification rates increase up to 35% in patients suffering from complex elbow injuries [37, 16]. Even though intraoperative radiation as well as postoperative NSAID therapy represent useful therapeutic options to prevent from excessive heterotopic ossifications [45], they are not recommended in treating Monteggia fractures in general. The use should rather be considered depending on fracture type and intraoperative trauma [16].

Nerve injuries with persisting nerve palsies are described in 2–9% of the patients [44]. Depending on the type of RH luxation (Bado type I vs. Bado type II) the anterior and posterior interosseous nerves are in danger due to their anatomically close relationship to the radial head and neck [39, 46–48]. Neurovascular compromise can also occur during closed reduction, followed by splinting the swollen elbow in 90–100° flexion [36]. Iatrogenic nerve injuries of the radial and ulnar nerve following operative treatment of complex Monteggia fractures are also described in current literature. Not least because of these different causes of potential nerve injuries, a preoperative well documented neurological assessment should be performed in any case [16].

The risk of developing a forearm compartment syndrome has to be considered especially in dislocated Monteggia fractures and Monteggia-like lesions with extended soft tissue involvement. Continuous controls of swelling, neurovascular status and pain is highly recommended to not miss this emergency complication [16].

References

1. Laun R, Wild M, Brosius L, Hakimi M. Monteggia-like lesions – treatment strategies and one-year results. GMS Interdiscip Plast Reconstr Surg DGPW. 2015;4:Doc13.
2. Korner J, Hoffmann A, Rudig L, et al. Monteggia injuries in adults: critical analysis of injury pattern, management, and results. Unfallchirurg. 2004;107(11):1026–40.
3. Bado JL. The Monteggia lesion. Clin Orthop Relat Res. 1967;50:71–86.
4. Suarez R, Barquet A, Fresco R. Epidemiology and treatment of Monteggia lesion in adults: series of 44 cases. Acta Ortop Bras. 2016;24(1):48–51.
5. Ring D, Jupiter JB, Waters PM. Monteggia fractures in children and adults. J Am Acad Orthop Surg. 1998;6(4):215–24.
6. Rehim SA, Maynard MA, Sebastin SJ, Chung KC. Monteggia fracture dislocations: a historical review. J Hand Surg Am. 2014;39(7):1384–94.
7. Jupiter JB, Leibovic SJ, Ribbans W, Wilk RM. The posterior Monteggia lesion. J Orthop Trauma. 1991;5(4):395–402.
8. Giannicola G, Sacchetti FM, Greco A, Cinotti G, Postacchini F. Management of complex elbow instability. Musculoskelet Surg. 2010;94(Suppl 1):S25–36.
9. Josten C, Freitag S. Monteggia and Monteggia-like-lesions: classification, indication, and techniques in operative treatment. Eur J Trauma Emerg Surg. 2009;35(3):296–304.
10. Konrad GG, Kundel K, Kreuz PC, Oberst M, Sudkamp NP. Monteggia fractures in adults: long-term results and prognostic factors. J Bone Joint Surg Br. 2007;89(3):354–60.
11. Greiwe. Shoulder and Elbow Trauma and its Complications. Cambridge: Woodhead Publishing; 2016.
12. Giannicola G, Greco A, Sacchetti FM, Cinotti G, Nofroni I, Postacchini F. Complex fracture-dislocations of the proximal ulna and radius in adults: a comprehensive classification. J Shoulder Elb Surg. 2011;20(8):1289–99.
13. Mouhsine E, Akiki A, Castagna A, et al. Transolecranon anterior fracture dislocation. J Shoulder Elb Surg. 2007;16(3):352–7.
14. Ring D, Jupiter JB, Sanders RW, Mast J, Simpson NS. Transolecranon fracture-dislocation of the elbow. J Orthop Trauma. 1997;11(8):545–50.
15. Bruce HE, Harvey JP, Wilson JC Jr. Monteggia fractures. J Bone Joint Surg Am. 1974;56(8):1563–76.
16. Lendemans S, Taeger G, Nast-Kolb D. Dislocation fractures of the forearm. Galeazzi, Monteggia, and Essex-Lopresti injuries. Unfallchirurg. 2008;111(12):1005–14. quiz 15-6

17. Giannicola G, Manauzzi E, Cinotti G. Management of bilateral complex fracture-dislocation of proximal ulna and radius: a case report. Musculoskelet Surg. 2012;96(Suppl 1):S87–92.
18. Johnston GW. A follow-up of one hundred cases of fracture of the head of the radius with a review of the literature. Ulster Med J. 1962;31:51–6.
19. van Riet RP, Morrey BF. Documentation of associated injuries occurring with radial head fracture. Clin Orthop Relat Res. 2008;466(1):130–4.
20. Hotchkiss RN. Displaced fractures of the radial head: internal fixation or excision? J Am Acad Orthop Surg. 1997;5(1):1–10.
21. Giannicola G, Scacchi M, Sacchetti FM, Cinotti G. Clinical usefulness of proximal ulnar and radial fracture-dislocation comprehensive classification system (PURCCS): prospective study of 39 cases. J Shoulder Elb Surg. 2013;22(12):1729–36.
22. Sandmann GH, Siebenlist S, Lenich A, et al. Traumatic elbow dislocations in bouldering. Unfallchirurg. 2014;117(3):274–80.
23. Morrey BF, An KN, Stormont TJ. Force transmission through the radial head. J Bone Joint Surg Am. 1988;70(2):250–6.
24. Lenich A, Siebenlist S. What to do with the acute elbow-instability? A treatment plan. MMW Fortschr Med. 2012;154(14):56–9.
25. Strauss EJ, Tejwani NC, Preston CF, Egol KA. The posterior Monteggia lesion with associated ulnohumeral instability. J Bone Joint Surg Br. 2006;88(1):84–9.
26. Beser CG, Demiryurek D, Ozsoy H, et al. Redefining the proximal ulna anatomy. Surg Radiol Anat. 2014;36(10):1023–31.
27. Wadia F, Kamineni S, Dhotare S, Amis A. Radiographic measurements of normal elbows: clinical relevance to olecranon fractures. Clin Anat. 2007;20(4):407–10.
28. Wang AA, Mara M, Hutchinson DT. The proximal ulna: an anatomic study with relevance to olecranon osteotomy and fracture fixation. J Shoulder Elb Surg. 2003;12(3):293–6.
29. Tompkins DG. The anterior Monteggia fracture: observations on etiology and treatment. J Bone Joint Surg Am. 1971;53(6):1109–14.
30. Penrose JH. The Monteggia fracture with posterior dislocation of the radial head. J Bone Joint Surg Br. 1951;33-B(1):65–73.
31. Mullick S. The lateral Monteggia fracture. J Bone Joint Surg Am. 1977;59(4):543–5.
32. Biberthaler P, Kanz KG, Siebenlist S. Elbow joint dislocation – important considerations for closed reduction. MMW Fortschr Med. 2015;157(9):50–2.
33. Jeon IH, Sanchez-Sotelo J, Zhao K, An KN, Morrey BM. The contribution of the coronoid and radial head to the stability of the elbow. J Bone Joint Surg Br. 2012;94(1):86–92.
34. Wegmann K, Engel K, Skouras E, et al. Reconstruction of Monteggia-like proximal ulna fractures using different fixation devices: a biomechanical study. Injury. 2016;47(8):1636–41.
35. Celli A, Marongiu MC, Fontana M, Celli L. The fracture-dislocation of the forearm – Monteggia and Essex-Lopresti lesions. In: Celli A, Celli L, Morrey BF, editors. Treatment of elbow lesions – new aspects in diagnosis and surgical techniques, vol. 1. New York: Springer; 2008. p. 113–26.
36. Bae DS. Successful strategies for managing Monteggia injuries. J Pediatr Orthop. 2016;36(4):67–70.
37. Korner J, Hansen M, Weinberg A, Hessmann M, Rommens PM. Monteggia fractures in childhood?Diagnosis and management in acute and chronic cases. European Journal of Trauma. 2004;30(6):361–70.
38. Ring D, Waters P. Operative fixation of Monteggia fractures in children. J Bone Joint Surg Br. 1996;78(5):734–9.
39. Parisi TJ, Jupiter JB. Fractures of the proximal radius and ulna: Monteggia injuries. In: Greiwe RM, editor. Shoulder and elbow trauma and its complications, vol. 2. 1st ed. San Diego: Elsevier; 2016. p. 193–223.
40. Lendemans S, Taeger G, Nast-Kolb D. Dislocation fractures of the forearm. Galeazzi, Monteggia, and Essex-Lopresti injuries. Unfallchirurg. 2008;111(12):1005–14. quiz 15-6
41. Josten C, Freitag S. Monteggia and Monteggia-like-lesions: classification, indication, and techniques in operative treatment. Eur J Trauma Emerg Surg. 2009;35(3):296–304.
42. Suarez R, Barquet A, Fresco R. Epidemiology and treatment of Monteggia lesion in adults: series of 44 cases. Acta Ortop Bras. 2016;24(1):48–51.
43. Schmidt CM, Mann D, Schnabel M. Elastic stable intramedullary nailing as alternative therapy for pediatric Monteggia fractures. Unfallchirurg. 2008;111(5):350–7.
44. Burkhart KJ, Gruszka D, Frohn S, Wegmann K, Rommens PM, Eicker CM, et al. Locking plate osteosynthesis of the radial head fractures : clinical and radiological results. Unfallchirurg. 2015;118(11):949–56.
45. Frosch KH, Knopp W, Dresing K, Langer C, Sturmer KM. A bipolar radial head prosthesis after comminuted radial head fractures: indications, treatment and outcome after 5 years. Unfallchirurg. 2003;106(5):367–73.
46. Meffert RH, Eden L, Jansen H. Monteggia- und Monteggia-ähnliche Verletzungen. Trauma und Berufskrankheit. 2015;17(1):22–31.
47. Heyd R, Strassmann G, Schopohl B, Zamboglou N. Radiation therapy for the prevention of heterotopic ossification at the elbow. J Bone and Joint Surg (Br). 2001;83:332–4.
48. Celli A, Celli L. Elbow surgical approaches. In: Celli A, Celli L, Morrey BF, editors. Treatment of elbow lesions – new aspects in diagnosis and surgical techniques, vol. 1. New York: Springer; 2008. p. 39–59.

Terrible Triad Injuries

7

Michael Hackl and Lars Peter Müller

Epidemiology

The estimated incidence of elbow dislocations is 5.21 per 100.000 persons per year. Thereby, the elbow represents the second most commonly dislocated joint following the shoulder joint [17, 26, 44]. Terrible triad injuries comprise only 8% of all elbow dislocations and, hence, can be considered rather rare injuries [35].

The mean age of patients at the time of injury is 45 years with the dominant arm being involved more frequently (60.8%) [4, 6, 11, 14–16, 27, 28, 34–36, 40, 47, 48, 51]. Terrible triad injuries occur more commonly in men than in women with a male-to-female ratio of approximately 1.7: 1 [4, 6, 11, 14–16, 27, 28, 34–36, 40, 47, 48, 51]. They are associated with sports activities in nearly half of all cases [44].

Especially in case of a high-energy trauma, concomitant injuries to the ipsilateral shoulder, forearm or wrist can occur [11, 14, 28, 48].

Classification

The terrible triad injury has first been described by Hotchkiss [1] in 1996 and is defined as a

- posterior elbow dislocation with concomitant
- radial head fracture and
- coronoid fracture

Radial Head Fracture

Radial head fractures are classified according to the modified Mason classification [3] (cross reference to chapter 5). Since the terrible triad injury represents a fracture-dislocation, all radial head fractures in this injury pattern are considered type IV fractures. The majority of radial head fractures in terrible triad injuries are displaced fractures. 51.1% are displaced two-part fractures (corresponding to Mason type II); 40.7% represent multi-fragmentary fractures (corresponding to Mason type III). Only 8.2% of radial head fractures in terrible triad injuries are non-displaced two-part fractures (corresponding to Mason type I) [4, 6, 11, 14, 15, 27, 28, 35, 39, 47, 48, 51].

Coronoid Fracture

In 1989, Regan and Morrey proposed a classification system for coronoid fractures depending on the amount of the coronoid involved [37]. Type I fractures are considered as avulsion fractures of the coronoid tip. Fractures classified as type II involve less than 50% of the coronoid; type III

M. Hackl (✉) · L. P. Müller
Department of Orthopedic and Trauma Surgery, University Hospital of Cologne, Cologne, Germany
e-mail: michael.hackl@uk-koeln.de

P. Biberthaler et al. (eds.), *Acute Elbow Trauma*, Strategies in Fracture Treatments,
https://doi.org/10.1007/978-3-319-97850-5_7

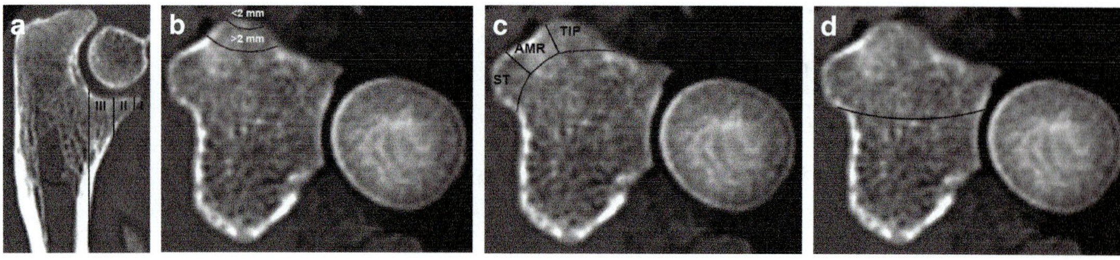

Fig. 7.1 Coronoid fracture classifications. (**a**) *Regan and Morrey classification*. *I*: avulsion of the *coronoid tip*; *II*: *<50%* of the coronoid height; *III*: *>50%* of the coronoid height [37]. (**b–d**) *O'Driscoll classification* [33]. (**b**) *I*: transverse shear fractures. *I.1*: <2 mm, *I.2*: >2 mm. (**c**) *II: anteromedial facet fractures*. *II.1*: anteromedial rim (AMR), *II.2*: AMR + coronoid tip (TIP), *II.3*: AMR + sublime tubercle (ST) ± tip. (**d**) *III*: basal fractures. *III.1*: coronoid body/base fractures, *III.2*: trans-olecranon basal coronoid fractures

fractures involve more than 50% of the coronoid process (Fig. 7.1a). Most coronoid fractures in terrible triad injuries are either type I (28.5%) or type II (68.9%). Type III fractures are rarely seen in terrible triad injuries and comprise only 2.6% of all cases [4, 6, 11, 14, 15, 27, 28, 35, 39, 47, 48, 51].

O'Driscoll formed a new classification system in 2003 which takes different fracture mechanisms into consideration: Type I fractures are transverse shear fractures (Fig. 7.1b). Type II fractures represent fractures of the anteromedial facet (Fig. 7.1c). Particularly type II.3 fractures, which involve the sublime tubercle, result in pronounced valgus and posteromedial instability. Type III fractures are fractures of the base or the body of the coronoid (Fig. 7.1d) [33]. Coronoid fractures in terrible triad injuries are usually transverse shear fractures according to O'Driscoll type I. Type II or III fractures are seldomly seen [8, 9, 14, 28, 51].

Symptoms and Diagnostics

Initial Evaluation

Patients with terrible triad injuries usually present immediately after trauma with painful swelling and tenderness of the elbow. The injury mechanism might not be remembered in detail, yet, most patients describe a fall on the outstretched hand. The injury commonly occurs due to high-energy trauma and/or during sports; particularly in elderly patients, a low-energy trauma can also result in terrible triad injuries. Deformity of the elbow may or may not be present as the elbow joint reduces spontaneously prior to presentation in some cases. A thorough physical examination is mandatory in order to evaluate any possible *concomitant injuries* – especially but not limited to the ipsilateral shoulder, forearm and wrist. Injuries to the skin must be inspected as they could be suggestive of an open fracture. The *neurovascular status* has to be obtained and documented.

Diagnostic Workup

First, conventional radiographs of the elbow in antero-posterior and lateral view have to be obtained. An additional oblique view can be useful to further evaluate the radial head. Fractures of the coronoid are easy to miss as the fragments might be overlapped by the distal humerus or by radial head fragments. Small, triangular-shaped fragments proximal to the coronoid or the absence of the distinctive shape of the coronoid tip can hint at a coronoid fracture on lateral radiographs (Fig. 7.2).

If a posterior dislocation of the elbow joint is confirmed with conventional radiographs, *closed reduction* under anesthesia should subsequently be performed. The forearm is supinated and distraction forces are applied while moving the

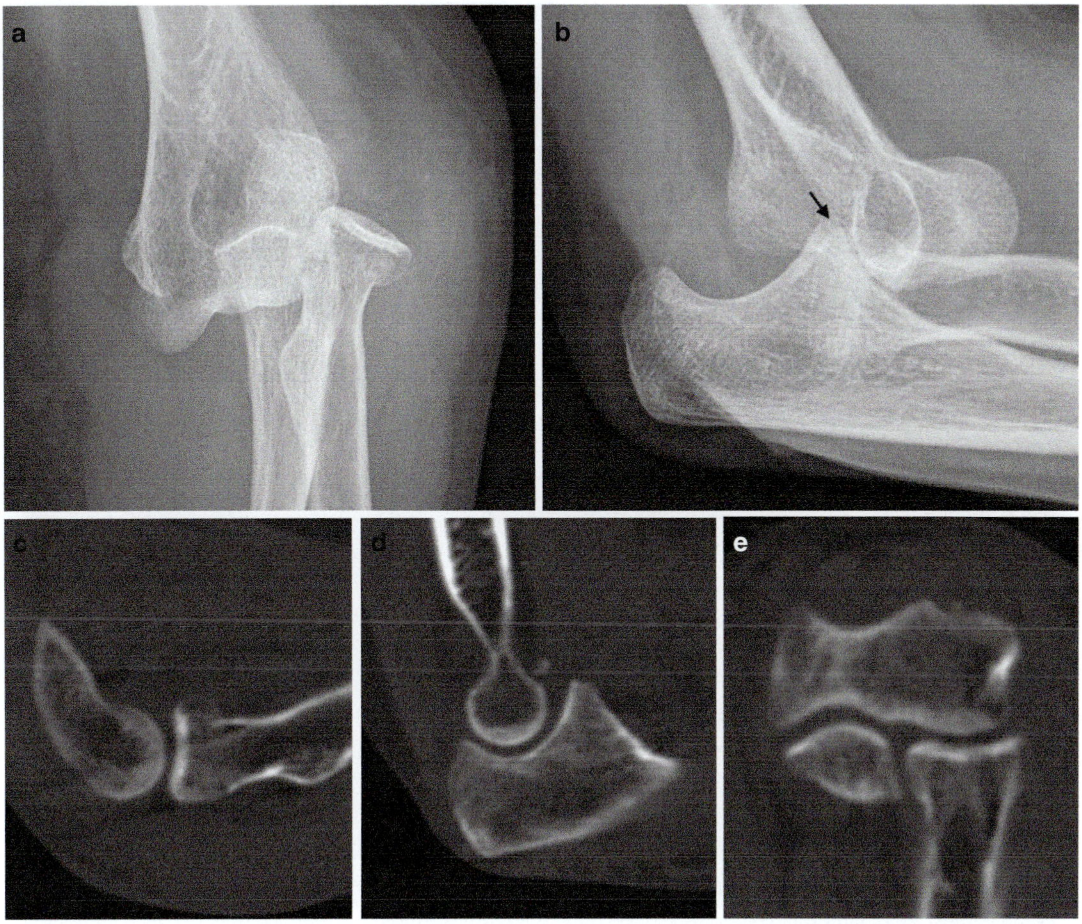

Fig. 7.2 Non-operative treatment of a terrible triad injury. (**a**, **b**) Plain radiographs upon presentation revealing a posterior elbow dislocation with radial neck fracture (Mason type II) and a coronoid tip fracture (O'Driscoll type I.1). The black arrow points to missing coronoid tip. (**c–e**) CT scans following closed reduction showing a concentric radiohumeral joint in a sagittal view (**c**), a concentric ulnohumeral joint in a sagittal view with displacement of the coronoid tip fragment (**d**) and a congruent joint in a coronal view (**e**)

elbow from extension to flexion in order to reduce the joint. Under fluoroscopy, varus and valgus stress tests should then be applied to evaluate the lateral and medial collateral ligament. The degree of valgus and varus instability should be documented. Moreover, the *joint stability* during passive flexion and extension has to be evaluated and documented. *Redislocation* during varus/valgus testing or upon flexion of the elbow joint of 30° or more is highly suspicious of gross instability. Immediately after joint reduction and evaluation of stability, a splint is applied in 90° of flexion and neutral rotation. The neurovascular status has to be obtained and documented again to rule out neurovascular complications.

Successful reduction has to be confirmed with standard radiographs. While standard radiographs may suffice in some cases, a subsequent computed tomography (CT) scan with three-dimensional reconstructions should be performed as it facilitates the fracture classification, the evaluation of joint congruity and the localization of displaced fragments (Figs. 7.2, 7.3, and 7.4). Additional magnetic resonance imag-

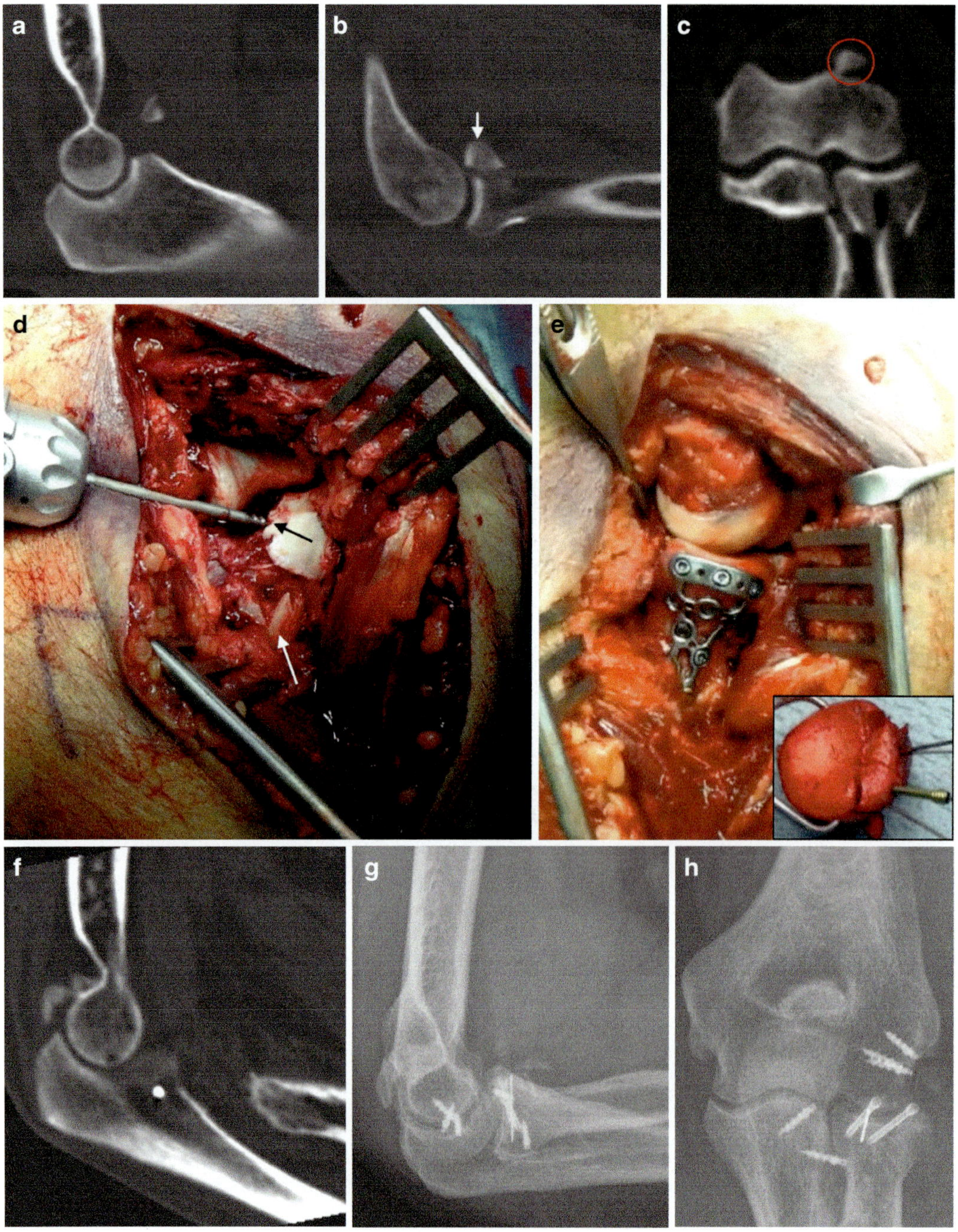

Fig. 7.3 Operative treatment of a terrible triad injury with ORIF of the radial head and suture anchor refixation of the coronoid tip. (**a**–**c**) Preoperative CT scans revealing a displaced coronoid fracture (O'Driscoll type I.2) (**a**) and a multi-fragmentary radial head fracture (**b**, **c**). The red circle (**c**) depicts a radial head fragment which lies at the posterior aspect of the capitulum as a result of the dislocation. (**d**, **e**) Intraoperative photographs. Lateral view through a Kocher approach. (**d**) After resection of the radial head fragments, suture anchor refixation of the coronoid tip (black arrow) is performed. The white arrow indicates the radial shaft. (**e**) After on-table reconstruction of the radial head (lower right corner), osteosynthesis of the radial head/neck fracture with an anatomically preshaped locking plate is performed. (**f**–**h**) CT scan and plain radiographs 1 year postoperatively showing a consolidated radial head fracture. In the meanwhile, removal of the plate has been performed. The CT scans and plain radiographs reveal heterotopic ossification (HO) in the olecranon fossa limiting extension. The patient was satisfied with the outcome and did not want to undergo revision for removal of the HO

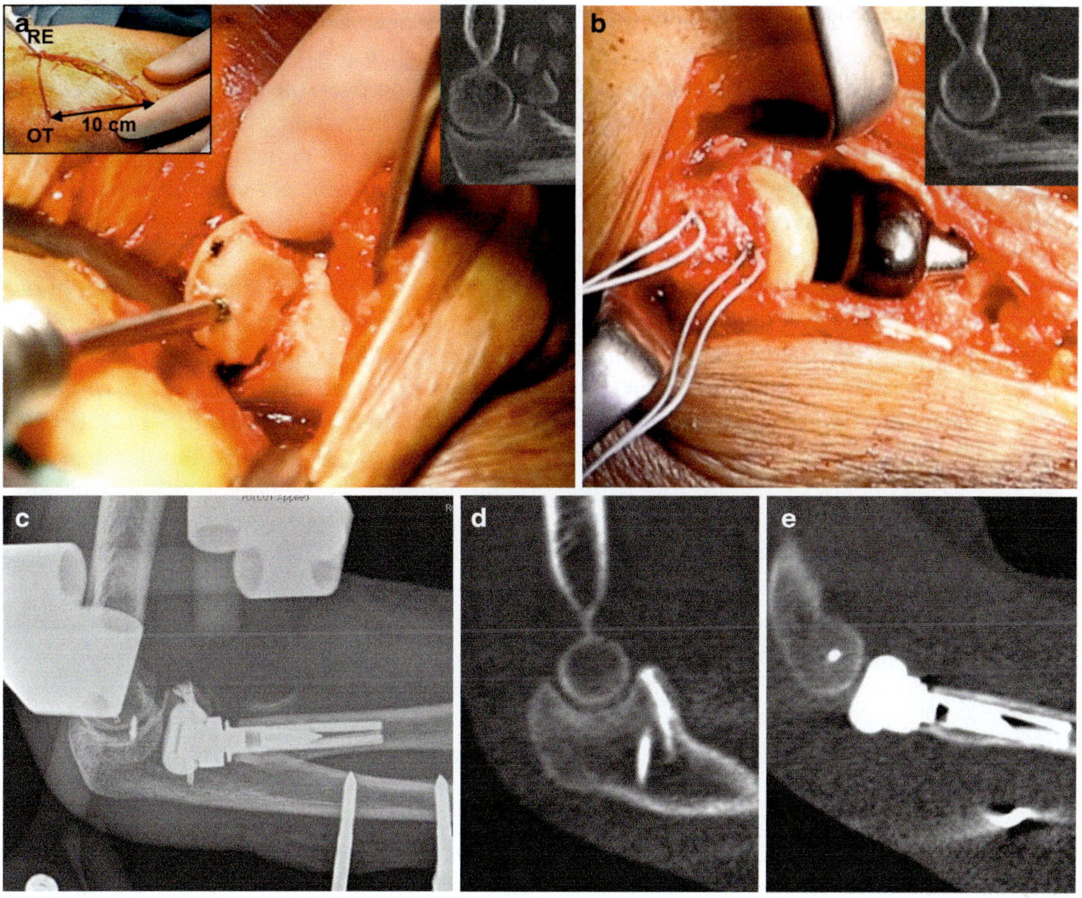

Fig. 7.4 Operative treatment of a terrible triad injury with radial head replacement and coronoid reconstruction. (**a**) Reconstruction of the coronoid with a radial head fragment. Left upper corner: Illustration of the skin incision – a rectangular triangle is drawn from the olecranon tip (OT) to the radial epicondyle (RE) and to a point 10 cm distal to the olecranon tip. The skin incision is performed over the hypotenuse of this triangle which serves as a projection of the Kocher interval. (**b**) Replacement of the radial head with a modular, monopolar radial head prosthesis. (**c**) Postoperative radiograph in the lateral view. Due to persistent instability after radial head replacement and coronoid reconstruction, a hinged external fixator was applied. (**d, e**) Joint congruity with consolidated coronoid reconstruction and intact radial head replacement at the latest follow-up

ing (MRI) of the elbow joint is usually not necessary.

Injury Pattern and Surgery Related Anatomy

Injury Mechanism

Terrible triad injuries typically occur due to a *fall on the outstretched hand* with the elbow extended or slightly bent. Fitzpatrick et al. [13] were able to show by means of an in-vitro biomechanical study that terrible triad injuries occur more frequently as a result of a fall on the *pronated forearm* while supination of the forearm typically leads to simple elbow dislocation. Pronation enforces joint congruity because of pre-tensioning of the lateral stabilizers [10, 24]. It might thus increase the osseous impact and increase the probability for radial head and/or coronoid fractures in posterior elbow dislocation.

As a result of the impact of the fall, the forearm rotates externally or internally and translates posteriorly which ultimately leads to posterior dislocation. The coronoid process and the "anterior rim" of the radial head act as primary constraints against posterior translation of the forearm. Hence, the coronoid process gets perched underneath the trochlea which leads to *transverse shearing fractures* of the coronoid (O'Driscoll type I [33]). Similarly, the "*anterior rim*" of the radial head hits against the capitulum causing a radial head fracture. Initial varus or valgus load causes radiocapitellar or ulnohumeral abutment which might result in more complex fractures of the radial head and/or the coronoid process. Especially in high-energy trauma, the axial compression forces may lead to multi-fragmentary radial head fractures and larger coronoid fractures.

Radial head fractures – and terrible triad injuries even more so – represent osteoligamentous injuries [23]. According to a study by McKee et al. [30], terrible triad injuries go along with *disruption of the lateral collateral ligament* (LCL) in 100% of cases while the *medial collateral ligament* (MCL) is disrupted in 56% of patients. The most common site of disruption for both the MCL and the LCL is their humeral origin [30].

Surgery Related Anatomy and Biomechanics

Along with the MCL, the radial head serves as the main *valgus stabilizer* of the elbow [45]. Moreover, approximately 60% of axial forces along the elbow joint are transmitted through the radial column – making the radial head a crucial *axial stabilizer* [32]. Consequently, radial head resection has a devastating effect on the stability of the elbow joint [2]. Particularly in case of concomitant osseous and ligamentous injuries – as present in terrible triad injuries – *radial head resection* is *obsolete* and the radial column has to be preserved. If reconstruction of the radial head is not feasible, radial head replacement should therefore be performed instead. Even though available radial head prostheses cannot completely reproduce the biomechanical profile of the native radial head, they restore valgus and axial stability [21, 41, 45]. In the acute setting, *monopolar prostheses* may be preferred over bipolar implants as they may provide superior radiocapitellar stability [5, 31].

Coronoid fractures increase rotatory instability of the elbow as the fractured coronoid can no longer act as a constraint against the trochlea when posterior translation forces are applied. Moreover, the coronoid can be considered as an important stabilizer against varus forces [22]. Open reduction and internal fixation (ORIF) of the coronoid is mandatory in type III fractures of the coronoid as well as in any fracture involving the *sublime tubercle* – which represents the attachment site of the MCL and therefore contributes to valgus stability of the elbow – and should at least be considered in type II fractures in order to sufficiently restore joint stability [42]. If ORIF of the coronoid is not possible due to severe comminution, the olecranon tip, a bone graft (harvested from the iliac crest) or a fragment of the fractured radial head should be used to reconstruct the coronoid (Fig. 7.4) [25].

Therapeutic Options

Non-operative Treatment

While the vast majority of terrible triad injuries require surgical treatment [29], some cases can be treated non-operatively [4, 15] if the following *criteria* are fulfilled (Fig. 7.2):

- joint congruity following closed reduction
- stable flexion arc without tendency to redislocate (extension lag <30°)
- minimally displaced radial head fracture (<2 mm corresponding to Mason type I [3])
- small transverse shear fracture of the coronoid (<30% of the coronoid process) without involvement of the anteromedial facet
- no block of motion upon flexion-extension and pronosupination (e.g. due to intra-articular osteochondral lesions)

A *close follow-up* of patients undergoing conservative treatment is mandatory. If one or more of the above-mentioned criteria are not being met any longer, surgical revision has to be considered.

In our clinical practice, the patient's elbow is immobilized in a *splint* at 90° of elbow flexion and neutral rotation for *7–10 days* before an early *functional treatment* regimen is initiated. A hinged elbow orthosis is then applied which allows flexion and extension in neutral rotation. Within the orthosis, extension is limited to 20° for 4 weeks to avoid full extension which could predispose to recurrent instability. Physical therapy should at least be performed two to three times a week. During physical therapy, the orthosis can be removed to carefully mobilize the joint over the full range of motion. Pronosupination should only be performed in 90° of flexion. Four weeks after trauma, static progressive splinting in extension maybe performed overnight to counteract flexion contracture. Load bearing is introduced at week 7 or after radiologic evidence of fracture consolidation.

Surgical Treatment

If any of the criteria for conservative therapy are not fulfilled and no absolute contraindications for surgery are present, operative treatment is recommended for terrible triad injuries to restore joint congruity and stability.

Diagnostic arthroscopy may be performed at the beginning of the surgery to evaluate the injuries or to retrieve displaced fragments especially from the posterior aspect of the elbow joint (Fig. 7.3c). In case of simple two-part fractures of the radial head (Mason type II) and the coronoid process (O'Driscoll type I, Regan and Morrey type I/II) without comminution, arthroscopically assisted, percutaneous reduction and internal fixation of the radial head and the coronoid can be attempted with cannulated headless compression screws. If this treatment strategy does not succeed or in case of a more severe fracture pattern – as common in terrible triad injuries –an open, lateral approach is indicated.

Lateral Approach

The patient is placed in *supine* position with the arm resting on an arm board in 90° of abduction. A tourniquet may or may not be used depending on the surgeon's preference. A rectangular triangle is now drawn from the olecranon tip to the radial epicondyle and to a point 10 cm distal of the olecranon tip at the posterior edge of the ulna (Fig. 7.4a) as a projection of the anconeus muscle. The skin incision is performed at the hypotenuse of this triangle reflecting the *Kocher* interval between the anconeus and the extensor carpi ulnaris. After careful dissection of the skin and the subcutaneous tissue, the forearm fascia is incised to identify the "fatty streak" of the aforementioned Kocher's interval. Through blunt dissection, the anconeus and the extensor carpi ulnaris can be separated to expose the lateral collateral ligament and the joint capsule. The annular ligament and the joint capsule are incised longitudinally to reveal the underlying radial head. The lateral collateral ligament complex and the common extensors can be sharply released from the lateral epicondyle and reflected ventrally to allow better exposure of the radiocapitellar joint as well as the coronoid. Particularly in high-energy trauma, the lateral approach to the joint may already be established once dissecting through the skin and subcutaneous tissue due to the severely disrupted soft tissue structures (Fig. 7.3d).

In case of simple, non-comminuted shearing fractures of the coronoid (O'Driscoll type I) and the "anterior rim" of the radial head (corresponding to Mason type II), a common extensor split may suffice to achieve fracture reduction.

Treatment of the Radial Head Fracture

Once the approach has been established, the radial head fracture is evaluated. In case of a two- or three-part fracture with solid fragments, ORIF with cannulated headless compression screws is usually sufficient. If severe comminution of the entire radial head is present, an *on-table reconstruction* of the fragments should be attempted. If the radial head can be reasonably reconstructed, subsequent internal fixation with an anatomically pre-shaped locking plate can be performed (Fig. 7.3e). Care has to be taken to place the plate at the "*safe zone*" of the radial head – if possible – to avoid radioulnar impingement with limitation of pronosupination [38]. In full supination, the plate should be fixed close to the posterior edge of the proximal radioulnar joint in order to respect the "safe zone".

Whenever reconstruction of the radial head is not feasible or more than 30% of the radial head are missing [43], *radial head replacement* is recommended in order to restore radiocapitellar stability (Fig. 7.4b). Radial head resection should not be performed in a fracture-dislocation as it potentially leads to gross joint instability. We advocate the use of monopolar radial head prostheses in acute fracture-dislocations as biomechanical evidence suggests that they might lead to superior joint stability when compared to bipolar prostheses [5, 31]. Especially in terrible triad injuries, correct placement of the radial head replacement is crucial [18]. Slight *over- or understuffing* can severely alter joint biomechanics and can lead to radiocapitellar and ulnohumeral impingement or to persisting joint instability [45]. Van Riet et al. were able to validate the posterolateral edge of the lesser sigmoid notch of the ulna as a point of reference [46]. Hence, in order to adequately restore the radial length, the radial head prosthesis should be in line with this anatomic landmark.

When reviewing the current literature, surgical treatment of radial head fractures in terrible triad injuries consists of radial head replacement in nearly two thirds of the cases while ORIF is performed in approximately one third of treated patients [4, 7, 11, 12, 14–16, 27, 28, 34–36, 39, 48, 50, 51].

Treatment of the Coronoid Fracture

In general, we recommend coronoid fixation whenever possible to *optimize joint stability*. Before performing fixation of the radial head, the coronoid can be visualized through external rotation of the forearm – particularly in case of complete disintegration of the radial head (Fig. 7.3d).

In *O'Driscoll type I.1 fractures*, the fragment is usually too small for screw fixation. Fixation of these fractures can be achieved with suture anchors. One or two *suture anchors* are placed in the fracture bed with their respective sutures grasping the anterior capsule attached to the fragment. Thereby, tying of the sutures leads to reduction of the coronoid fragment. Alternatively, a *lasso loop* technique can be used where a suture is looped around the ulna through two anteroposterior drill holes and passed through the anterior capsule to, once again, achieve fracture reduction by tying the suture [36].

Screw or plate osteosynthesis is commonly used for *O'Driscoll type I.2 fractures*. If sufficient exposure of the coronoid is achieved through an extended Kocher approach, two K-wires can be placed through the proximal ulna from anterior to posterior for temporary fixation of the coronoid fragment. Two *cannulated headless compressions screws* can then be placed over the K-wires to reach stable internal fixation. Alternatively, plate osteosynthesis can be performed. In case of limited exposure of the coronoid, percutaneous placement of two K-wires from posterior to anterior can be used to achieve temporary fixation of the coronoid fracture with subsequent retrograde osteosynthesis with cannulated headless compression screws. In high-energy trauma, refixation of the coronoid fracture might not be feasible due to severe comminution. In that case, *reconstruction of the coronoid* can be performed with a radial head fragment – if the radial head has to be replaced at the same time – (Fig. 7.4a), with the tip of the olecranon or with a bone graft from the iliac crest.

In *O'Driscoll type II and type III fractures* – which are rarely seen in terrible triad injuries – plate osteosynthesis through an *additional medial approach* should be considered to achieve stable fracture fixation. As the coronoid can usually be exposed adequately through a lateral or medial approach, an anterior approach performing a brachialis split is obsolete used due to its close proximity to the neurovascular bundle.

LCL Repair

Following stable fixation of the radial head and the coronoid process, the lateral collateral ligament – along with the common extensors – has to be reattached to its humeral original. We prefer placing one *suture anchor* into the motion axis of the capitulum for refixation of the lateral collateral ligament and another suture anchor in the lateral epicondyle for refixation of the common extensors (Fig. 7.4b). The *forearm fascia* has to be closed carefully as it contributes to lateral elbow stability and serves as an important barrier for deep infection.

Additional Procedures

Following ORIF of the radial head and the coronoid as well as reconstruction of the lateral soft tissue structures, joint stability should be evaluated once more. If valgus stability persists, an *additional medial approach* with refixation of the medial collateral ligament and the flexor-pronator mass has to be considered. Through a flexor carpi ulnaris split, the decompression of the ulnar nerve can be performed and the medial collateral ligament as well as the flexor-pronator mass arising from the medial epicondyle can be exposed. Analogical to the lateral approch, refixation of the medial soft tissue structures can be performed by *suture anchoring*.

Instead of or in addition to medial repair, a *hinged external fixator* can be applied if persisting instability is present. Great care has to be taken to place the hinge of the external fixator in line with the motion axis of elbow joint to achieve concentric flexion and extension. The guide wire can be placed in the lateral epicondyle before wound closure. This facilitates the correct positioning of the guide wire due to better exposure. Placement of the humeral pins has to be performed cautiously in order to avoid radial nerve injuries [19, 20, 49]. We recommend a mini-open approach through a small incision to minimize the risk of neurological complications.

Alternatively to the described protocol, some surgeons prefer a *posterior longitudinal skin incision* establishing full-thickness flaps around the elbow to be able to approach the joint laterally and medially through a single incision.

Figure 7.5 summarizes the aforementioned *treatment algorithm* for terrible triad injuries.

Postoperative Care

Following surgical treatment, elastic compression bandages are applied until swelling subsides. The patient's arm is placed in a hinged elbow orthosis which limits extension to 20° for 4 weeks and flexion to 90° for the first week. Afterwards, flexion is increased by 10° each week. Within the orthosis, the patient can actively flex and extend the elbow in neutral rotation within the described range of motion. Physical therapy can be introduced immediately after surgery. During physical therapy, the orthosis can be removed to perform active-assistive flexion and extension over the full range of motion. Pronosupination should be performed at 90° of flexion only. At week 5, static progressive splinting in extension can be introduced overnight to avoid flexion contracture. The orthosis is usually removed after 6 weeks. Load bearing is introduced at week 7 or after radiologic evidence of fracture consolidation.

If a hinged external fixator had to be applied, the hinge initially remains blocked. After 7 days, the hinge is released and active flexion and extension can be performed. The external fixator is removed after 6 weeks but can be applied for up to twelve weeks if there is pronounced instability.

Outcomes and Complications

Non-operative Treatment

Only few patients meet the presented criteria for non-operative treatment of terrible triad injuries. According to McKee et al. [29], *less than 5%* of patients with terrible triad injuries can undergo non-operative treatment. Thus, only few reports of conservative therapy are available in the literature. Guitton et al. [15] reported a case series of four patients who underwent non-operative treatment following posterior elbow dislocation with associated radial head and coronoid fractures. While three of their patients had good to excellent clinical results at the latest follow-up, one 32-year old male patient developed ulnar neuropathy and had to undergo revision surgery 8 months after trauma. This patient had a Mason type II fracture with more than 5 mm of displacement involving about 30% of the articular surface and thus did not meet the presented criteria for non-operative treatment (check algorithm – Fig. 7.5).

In 2014, Chan et al. [4] reported so far the largest case series of 12 patients who underwent non-operative therapy following a terrible triad

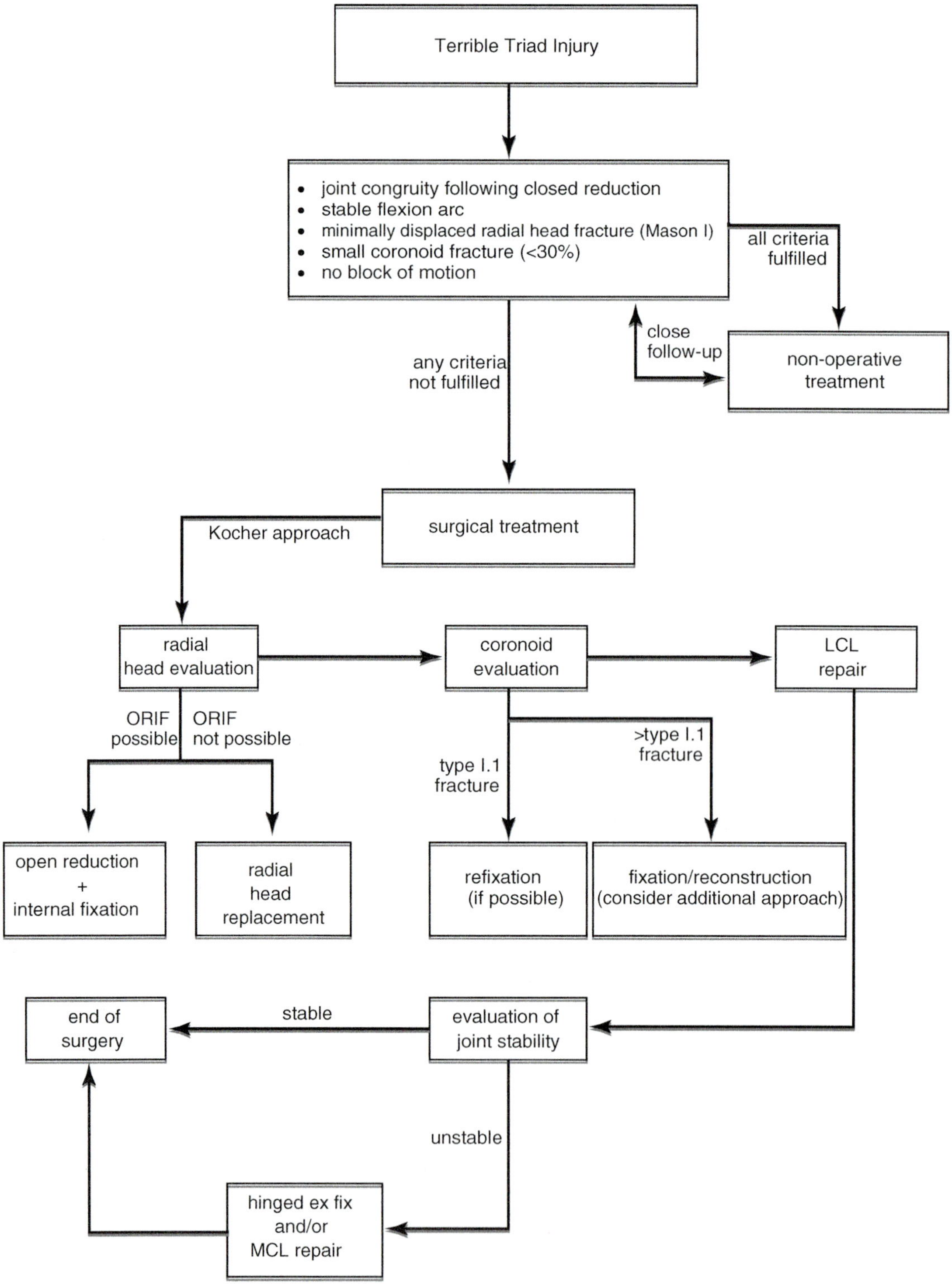

Fig. 7.5 Treatment algorithm for terrible triad injuries

injury. At a mean follow-up of 36 months, their patients had a mean flexion arc of 128° with a mean flexion contracture of 6°. The Mayo Elbow Performance Score averaged 94 out of 100 points and the mean Disabilities of the Arm, Shoulder and Hand (DASH) Score was 8 points. Two of their patients experienced complications: One patient had to undergo revision for early recurrent instability. Another had arthroscopic debridement for heterotopic ossification in the olecranon fossa. The study of Chan et al. [4] shows that non-operative treatment can lead to excellent clinical outcome when correctly indicated.

Surgical Treatment (Table 7.1)

The Early Stages

Early reports of surgical treatment for terrible triad injuries did not contain a standardized treatment protocol. Subsequently, Ring et al. reported poor results in seven of their eleven cases back in 2002 [40]. In none of the cases did they perform coronoid fixation and in four cases the radial head was resected which might explain their unsatisfactory results [40].

Establishing Standardized Protocols

Consequently, Pugh et al. [36] described a *standardized protocol* that is still considered valid today containing of a lateral Kocher approach, radial head reconstruction or replacement, coronoid fixation and lateral collateral ligament repair. If instability persisted following these procedures, the authors suggested medial collateral ligament repair and/or the use of a hinged external fixator. After a mean of 34 months, they reported a mean Mayo Elbow Performance Score of 88 points in their 36 patients. The flexion arc averaged 112° ± 11°. Eight of their patients (22%) had to undergo revision surgery for elbow stiffness (4), synostosis (2), infection (1) and recurrent instability (1) [36]. While their treatment protocol improved the overall clinical outcome significantly, complications following this severe injury remain fairly common.

Doing It Right the First Time

Initial correct treatment of terrible triad injuries is crucial in order to minimize the risk of lasting disability. Lindenhovius et al. [28] were able to show that patients who initially underwent inadequate treatment went on to have worse clinical

Table 7.1 Clinical outcome following surgical treatment of terrible triad injuries

Author	Year	n	FU	RH	Coronoid fixation	Other	Rom	Score	Compl.
Ring et al. [40]	2002	11	84	5 ORIF, 4 resection, 2 none	0/11	none	n/a	BMS: 76	7/11
Pugh et al. [36]	2004	36	34	20 ORIF, 13 RHR, 3 none	36/36	2 hinged ex fix	112°	MEPS: 88	8/36
Egol et al. [11]	2007	29	27	8 ORIF, 15 RHR, 3 resection	0/29	13 hinged ex fix	109°	MEPS: 81, DASH: 28	13/29
Forthman et al. [14]	2007	22	28	1 ORIF, 20 RHR, 1 allograft	22/22	4 ulnar nerve release	112°	MEPS: 86, DASH: 13	8/22
Lindenhovius et al. [28]	2008	18	29	1 ORIF, 17 RHR	18/18	4 ulnar nerve release	119°	MEPS: 88, DASH: 15	5/18
Leigh et al. [27]	2012	24	41	13 ORIF, 11 RHR	23/23	none	135°	ASES: 85, DASH: 10	7/24
Watters et al. [48]	2013	39	24	9 ORIF, 30 RHR	39/39	none	115°	BMS: 90, DASH: 16	14/39
Zhang et al. [51]	2014	21	32	19 ORIF, 2 RHR	21/21	none	126°	MEPS: 95	5/21

A review of literature

n number of cases, *FU* follow-up time, *RH* radial head, *Rom* range of motion, *Compl.* complications, *ORIF* open reduction and internal fixation, *RHR* radial head replacement, *ex fix* external fixator, *BMS* broberg-morrey score, *MEPS* mayo elbow performance score, *DASH* disabilities of the arm, shoulder and hand score outcomes despite revision (subacute cohort) than patients who were treated acutely (acute cohort). The acute cohort had a mean flexion arc of 119° with an average flexion contracture of 17° while the subacute cohort had a mean range of motion of only 100° with an average extension lag of 30° ($p < .05$).

ORIF vs Radial Head Arthroplasty

Two studies have focused on the influence of ORIF versus replacement of the radial head regarding the clinical results following terrible triad injuries. Watters et al. [48] did not observe any significant differences between groups in terms of range of motion as well as DASH and Broberg/Morrey scores at a minimum of 18 months follow-up. However, *radiographic signs of osteoarthritis* were seen more frequently in patients who underwent radial head arthroplasty. On the other hand, patients who underwent *ORIF were revised more frequently* (4/9) than patients who had radial head replacement (7/30). Due to a limited amount of cases, no significant differences could be obtained. Similarly, Leigh et al. [27] found that revision surgery was more common in the ORIF group (5/13) than in the radial head replacement group (2/11) after a mean follow-up of 41 months.

Systematic Review

A systematic review of available data regarding the outcome of terrible triad injuries reveals a *mean flexion arc of 113°* with an average flexion contracture of 18° and a mean pronosupination of 138°. The mean DASH score was 17 points, the Mayo Elbow Performance and Broberg/Morrey score averaged 87 points at the latest follow-up [4, 7, 11, 12, 14–16, 27, 28, 34–36, 39, 48, 50, 51]. *Elbow stiffness* represents the most common complication following terrible triad injuries and can be observed in 10.3% of all cases. *Failure of osteosynthesis* was found to be the second most common complication with 6.7%, followed by *ulnar neuropathy* (6.2%). *Recurrent instability* was seen in 2.6% while complications related to the radial head replacement – mostly due to *overstuffing* – were found in 1.9%. Treatment of terrible triad injuries was complicated by *infection* in 1.2% of cases [4, 7, 11, 12, 14–16, 27, 28, 34–36, 39, 48, 50, 51]. Heterotopic ossification and radiographic signs of osteoarthritis are common following terrible triad injuries but only rarely influence the clinical results [7].

References

1. Hotchkiss RN. Fractures and dislocations of the elbow. In: Rockwood CA Jr., Green DP, Bucholz RW, Heckman JD, eds. Rockwood and green's fractures in adults. Philadelphia, PA. Lippincott-Raven 1996;929–1024.
2. Beingessner DM, Dunning CE, Gordon KD, Johnson JA, King GJ. The effect of radial head excision and arthroplasty on elbow kinematics and stability. J Bone Joint Surg Am. 2004;86-A:1730–9.
3. Broberg MA, Morrey BF. Results of treatment of fracture-dislocations of the elbow. Clin Orthop Relat Res. 1987;216:109–19.
4. Chan K, MacDermid JC, Faber KJ, King GJ, Athwal GS. Can we treat select terrible triad injuries nonoperatively? Clin Orthop Relat Res. 2014;472:2092–9. https://doi.org/10.1007/s11999-014-3518-9.
5. Chanlalit C, Shukla DR, Fitzsimmons JS, An KN, O'Driscoll SW. The biomechanical effect of prosthetic design on radiocapitellar stability in a terrible triad model. J Orthop Trauma. 2012;26:539–44. https://doi.org/10.1097/BOT.0b013e318238b3a2.
6. Chen HW, Liu GD, Ou S, Fei J, Zhao GS, Wu LJ, et al. Operative treatment of terrible triad of the elbow via posterolateral and anteromedial approaches. PLoS One. 2015;10:e0124821. https://doi.org/10.1371/journal.pone.0124821.
7. Chen HW, Liu GD, Wu LJ. Complications of treating terrible triad injury of the elbow: a systematic review. PLoS One. 2014;9:e97476. https://doi.org/10.1371/journal.pone.0097476.
8. Doornberg JN, Ring D. Coronoid fracture patterns. J Hand Surg Am. 2006;31:45–52. https://doi.org/10.1016/j.jhsa.2005.08.014.
9. Doornberg JN, van Duijn J, Ring D. Coronoid fracture height in terrible-triad injuries. J Hand Surg Am. 2006;31:794–7. https://doi.org/10.1016/j.jhsa.2006.01.004.
10. Dunning CE, Zarzour ZD, Patterson SD, Johnson JA, King GJ. Muscle forces and pronation stabilize the lateral ligament deficient elbow. Clin Orthop Relat Res. 2001;388:118–24.
11. Egol KA, Immerman I, Paksima N, Tejwani N, Koval KJ. Fracture-dislocation of the elbow functional outcome following treatment with a standardized protocol. Bull NYU Hosp Jt Dis. 2007;65:263–70.
12. Fitzgibbons PG, Louie D, Dyer GS, Blazar P, Earp B. Functional outcomes after fixation of "terrible triad" elbow fracture disloca-

tions. Orthopedics. 2014;37:e373–6. https://doi.org/10.3928/01477447-20,140,401-59.
13. Fitzpatrick MJ, Diltz M, McGarry MH, Lee TQ. A new fracture model for "terrible triad" injuries of the elbow: influence of forearm rotation on injury patterns. J Orthop Trauma. 2012;26:591–6. https://doi.org/10.1097/BOT.0b013e31824135af.
14. Forthman C, Henket M, Ring DC. Elbow dislocation with intra-articular fracture: the results of operative treatment without repair of the medial collateral ligament. J Hand Surg Am. 2007;32:1200–9. https://doi.org/10.1016/j.jhsa.2007.06.019.
15. Guitton TG, Ring D. Nonsurgically treated terrible triad injuries of the elbow: report of four cases. J Hand Surg Am. 2010;35:464–7. https://doi.org/10.1016/j.jhsa.2009.12.015.
16. Gupta A, Barei D, Khwaja A, Beingessner D. Single-staged treatment using a standardized protocol results in functional motion in the majority of patients with a terrible triad elbow injury. Clin Orthop Relat Res. 2014;472:2075–83. https://doi.org/10.1007/s11999-014-3475-3.
17. Hackl M, Beyer F, Wegmann K, Leschinger T, Burkhart KJ, Muller LP. The treatment of simple elbow dislocation in adults. Dtsch Arztebl Int. 2015;112:311–9. https://doi.org/10.3238/arztebl.2015.0311.
18. Hackl M, Burkhart KJ, Wegmann K, Hollinger B, Lichtenberg S, Muller LP. From radial head to radiocapitellar to total elbow replacement: a case report. Int J Surg Case Rep. 2015;15:35–8. https://doi.org/10.1016/j.ijscr.2015.08.015.
19. Hackl M, Damerow D, Leschinger T, Scaal M, Muller LP, Wegmann K. Radial nerve location at the posterior aspect of the humerus: an anatomic study of 100 specimens. Arch Orthop Trauma Surg. 2015;135:1527–32. https://doi.org/10.1007/s00402-015-2300-0.
20. Hackl M, Lappen S, Burkhart KJ, Neiss WF, Muller LP, Wegmann K. The course of the median and radial nerve across the elbow: an anatomic study. Arch Orthop Trauma Surg. 2015;135:979–83. https://doi.org/10.1007/s00402-015-2228-4,
21. Hackl M, Wegmann K, Helf C, Neiss WF, Müller LP, Burkhart KJ. Die Passgenauigkeit monopolarer Radiuskopfprothesen im proximalen Radioulnargelenk. Obere Extremität. 2015;10:246–51. https://doi.org/10.1007/s11678-015-0337-x.
22. Hartzler RU, Llusa-Perez M, Steinmann SP, Morrey BF, Sanchez-Sotelo J. Transverse coronoid fracture: when does it have to be fixed? Clin Orthop Relat Res. 2014;472:2068–74. https://doi.org/10.1007/s11999-014-3477-1.
23. Itamura J, Roidis N, Mirzayan R, Vaishnav S, Learch T, Shean C. Radial head fractures: MRI evaluation of associated injuries. J Shoulder Elbow Surg. 2005;14:421–4. https://doi.org/10.1016/j.jse.2004.11.003.
24. Jensen SL, Olsen BS, Seki A, Ole Sojbjerg J, Sneppen O. Radiohumeral stability to forced translation: an experimental analysis of the bony constraint. J Shoulder Elbow Surg. 2002;11:158–65. https://doi.org/10.1067/mse.2002.121765.
25. Kataoka T, Moritomo H, Miyake J, Murase T, Sugamoto K. Three-dimensional suitability assessment of three types of osteochondral autograft for ulnar coronoid process reconstruction. J Shoulder Elbow Surg. 2014;23:143–50. https://doi.org/10.1016/j.jse.2013.10.004.
26. Kroner K, Lind T, Jensen J. The epidemiology of shoulder dislocations. Arch Orthop Trauma Surg. 1989;108:288–90.
27. Leigh WB, Ball CM. Radial head reconstruction versus replacement in the treatment of terrible triad injuries of the elbow. J Shoulder Elbow Surg. 2012;21:1336–41. https://doi.org/10.1016/j.jse.2012.03.005.
28. Lindenhovius AL, Jupiter JB, Ring D. Comparison of acute versus subacute treatment of terrible triad injuries of the elbow. J Hand Surg Am. 2008;33:920–6. https://doi.org/10.1016/j.jhsa.2008.02.007.
29. McKee MD, Pugh DM, Wild LM, Schemitsch EH, King GJ. Standard surgical protocol to treat elbow dislocations with radial head and coronoid fractures. Surgical technique. J Bone Joint Surg Am. 2005;87(Suppl 1):22–32. https://doi.org/10.2106/JBJS.D.02933.
30. McKee MD, Schemitsch EH, Sala MJ, O'Driscoll SW. The pathoanatomy of lateral ligamentous disruption in complex elbow instability. J Shoulder Elbow Surg. 2003;12:391–6. https://doi.org/10.1016/mse.2003.S1058274603000272.
31. Moon JG, Berglund LJ, Zachary D, An KN, O'Driscoll SW. Radiocapitellar joint stability with bipolar versus monopolar radial head prostheses. J Shoulder Elbow Surg. 2009;18:779–84. https://doi.org/10.1016/j.jse.2009.02.011.
32. Morrey BF, An KN, Stormont TJ. Force transmission through the radial head. J Bone Joint Surg Am. 1988;70:250–6.
33. O'Driscoll SW, Jupiter JB, Cohen MS, Ring D, McKee MD. Difficult elbow fractures: pearls and pitfalls. Instr Course Lect. 2003;52:113–34.
34. Papatheodorou LK, Rubright JH, Heim KA, Weiser RW, Sotereanos DG. Terrible triad injuries of the elbow: does the coronoid always need to be fixed? Clin Orthop Relat Res. 2014;472:2084–91. https://doi.org/10.1007/s11999-014-3471-7.
35. Pierrart J, Begue T, Mansat P, Geec. Terrible triad of the elbow: treatment protocol and outcome in a series of eighteen cases. Injury. 2015;46(Suppl 1):S8–S12. https://doi.org/10.1016/S0020-1383(15)70004-5.
36. Pugh DM, Wild LM, Schemitsch EH, King GJ, McKee MD. Standard surgical protocol to treat elbow dislocations with radial head and coronoid fractures. J Bone Joint Surg Am. 2004;86-A:1122–30.
37. Regan W, Morrey B. Fractures of the coronoid process of the ulna. J Bone Joint Surg Am. 1989;71:1348–54.
38. Ries C, Muller M, Wegmann K, Pfau DB, Muller LP, Burkhart KJ. Is an extension of the safe zone possible without jeopardizing the proximal radioulnar joint when performing a radial head plate osteosynthesis? J Shoulder Elbow Surg. 2015;24:1627–34. https://doi.org/10.1016/j.jse.2015.03.010.

39. Ring D, Hannouche D, Jupiter JB. Surgical treatment of persistent dislocation or subluxation of the ulnohumeral joint after fracture-dislocation of the elbow. J Hand Surg Am. 2004;29:470–80. https://doi.org/10.1016/j.jhsa.2004.01.005.
40. Ring D, Jupiter JB, Zilberfarb J. Posterior dislocation of the elbow with fractures of the radial head and coronoid. J Bone Joint Surg Am. 2002;84-A:547–51.
41. Sahu D, Holmes DM, Fitzsimmons JS, Thoreson AR, Berglund LJ, An KN, et al. Influence of radial head prosthetic design on radiocapitellar joint contact mechanics. J Shoulder Elbow Surg. 2014;23:456–62. https://doi.org/10.1016/j.jse.2013.11.028.
42. Schneeberger AG, Sadowski MM, Jacob HA. Coronoid process and radial head as posterolateral rotatory stabilizers of the elbow. J Bone Joint Surg Am. 2004;86-A:975–82.
43. Shukla DR, Thoreson AR, Fitzsimmons JS, An KN, O'Driscoll SW. The effect of capitellar impaction fractures on radiocapitellar stability. J Hand Surg Am. 2015;40:520–5. https://doi.org/10.1016/j.jhsa.2014.10.031.
44. Stoneback JW, Owens BD, Sykes J, Athwal GS, Pointer L, Wolf JM. Incidence of elbow dislocations in the United States population. J Bone Joint Surg Am. 2012;94:240–5. https://doi.org/10.2106/JBJS.J.01663.
45. Van Glabbeek F, Van Riet RP, Baumfeld JA, Neale PG, O'Driscoll SW, Morrey BF, et al. Detrimental effects of overstuffing or understuffing with a radial head replacement in the medial collateral-ligament deficient elbow. J Bone Joint Surg Am. 2004;86-A:2629–35.
46. van Riet RP, van Glabbeek F, de Weerdt W, Oemar J, Bortier H. Validation of the lesser sigmoid notch of the ulna as a reference point for accurate placement of a prosthesis for the head of the radius: a cadaver study. J Bone Joint Surg Br. 2007;89:413–6. https://doi.org/10.1302/0301-620X.89B3.18099.
47. Wang W, Liu JJ, Liu S, Ruan HJ, Li XJ, Fan CY. Arthrolysis combined with reconstruction for treatment of terrible triad injury with a poor outcome after surgical as well as conservative intervention. Arch Orthop Trauma Surg. 2014;134:325–31. https://doi.org/10.1007/s00402-014-1923-x.
48. Watters TS, Garrigues GE, Ring D, Ruch DS. Fixation versus replacement of radial head in terrible triad: is there a difference in elbow stability and prognosis? Clin Orthop Relat Res. 2014;472:2128–35. https://doi.org/10.1007/s11999-013-3331-x.
49. Wegmann K, Lappen S, Pfau DB, Neiss WF, Muller LP, Burkhart KJ. Course of the radial nerve in relation to the center of rotation of the elbow–the need for a rational safe zone for lateral pin placement. J Hand Surg Am. 2014;39:1136–40. https://doi.org/10.1016/j.jhsa.2014.03.019.
50. Zeiders GJ, Patel MK. Management of unstable elbows following complex fracture-dislocations–the "terrible triad" injury. J Bone Joint Surg Am. 2008;90(Suppl 4):75–84. https://doi.org/10.2106/JBJS.H.00893.
51. Zhang C, Zhong B, Luo CF. Treatment strategy of terrible triad of the elbow: experience in Shanghai 6th People's Hospital. Injury. 2014;45:942–8. https://doi.org/10.1016/j.injury.2013.12.012.

8 Varia: Distal Biceps Tendon Rupture

Arne Buchholz and Sebastian Siebenlist

Epidemiology

With an incidence of 3% of all biceps tendon injuries, the rupture of the distal biceps tendon is a rare injury. The most common site of injury of the distal biceps tendon is the avulsion from the radial tuberosity. Myotendinous or intratendinous injuries are uncommon. The majority of these ruptures affect almost exclusively physically active male patients between the ages of 30 and 60 years. The most common mechanism of injury involves eccentric muscle contraction against a heavy load applied to a flexed elbow. A recent epidemiological analysis revised the incidence upwards from 1.2/100,000 to 2.55/100.000 persons per year. They also evaluated risk factors related to rupture and found that smoking and elevated body mass index are associated with increased likelihood of injury [1, 2]. Other significant risk factors include anabolic steroid use and weightlifting [3, 4].

However the definitive pathogenesis of distal biceps tendon ruptures is not well understood. Both hypovascular and mechanical mechanisms seem to be responsible for tears. An anatomic study could show that there is a hypovascular zone approximately 2 cm proximal to the insertion on the radial tuberosity [5]. This watershed area could predispose the distal biceps tendon to rupture. Furthermore the study cited above evaluated radiologically the space available for the distal biceps tendon at the proximal radioulnar joint depending to forearm position. In moving from full forearm supination to pronation the space decreases by 50%, possibly leading to mechanical impingement of the tendon.

Symptoms and Diagnostics

Patients with a rupture of the distal biceps tendon often report a popping sound followed by acute pain in the antecubital fossa and an immediate weakness of elbow flexion and especially forearm supination. Swelling and hematoma may occur in different manifestations but are not obligatory. A loss of the normal biceps contour and a proximalization of the muscle belly may be present. However despite this presentation, a rupture may still be missed clinically, particularly when the lacertus fibrosus remains intact. Delayed diagnosis may defer primary reconstruction or lead to chronic weakness. The "squeeze-" and "hook test" are helpful physical exam maneuvers to detect reliably distal biceps ruptures

A. Buchholz
Clinic for Trauma Surgery, University Hospital Klinikum Rechts der Isar, Technical University, Munich, Germany
e-mail: arne.buchholz@mri.tum.de

S. Siebenlist (✉)
Department of Orthopaedic Sports Medicine, Technical University Munich Klinikum rechts der Isar, Munich, Germany
e-mail: sebastian.siebenlist@tum.de

P. Biberthaler et al. (eds.), *Acute Elbow Trauma*, Strategies in Fracture Treatments,
https://doi.org/10.1007/978-3-319-97850-5_8

[6, 7]. Analogous to the Thompson test for Achilles tendon ruptures, with the squeeze-test the muscle belly is firmly squeezed in 90° elbow flexion. The lack of forearm supination signifies a positive test. Ruland et al. found a sensitivity of 96% in diagnosing distal biceps ruptures with this test [6]. The hook-test is performed by inserting the index finger under the lateral edge of the biceps tendon in the antecubital fossa with the patients elbow flexed to 90° and the forearm fully supinated (Fig. 8.1). With an intact tendon, the examiner should be able to hook the finger about 1 cm deep under the resistant cord-like structure spanning the antecubital fossa. It is important to carry out the hook test from the lateral side to avoid mistaking the lacertus aponeurosis for an intact biceps tendon. O'Driscoll et al. showed a 100% sensitivity and specifity, that were higher than the sensitivity and specifity found with magnetic resonance imaging [7].

In terms of imaging, radiographs are usually obtained to rule out any associated elbow injuries, and occasionally show irregular changes about the radial tuberosity or an avulsion of the radial tuberosity itself. Ultrasound is a fast and cost-effective method that can confirm the clinical indications but it is user dependent [8]. Especially in partial rupture of the distal biceps tendon with an intact laceratus fibrosus, the clinical appearance is often less characteristic and the diagnosis may be difficult. In this caces advanced imaging should be performed out using MRI. Giuffre and Moss described the optimal patient position for magnetic resonance imaging of the distal biceps tendon; the flexed abducted supinated (FABS) position [9]. With the patient prone, shoulder abducted overhead, with elbow flexed to 90°, and forearm fully supinated, the full length of the biceps from the musculotendinous junction to the radial tuberosity insertion can be adequately demonstrated.

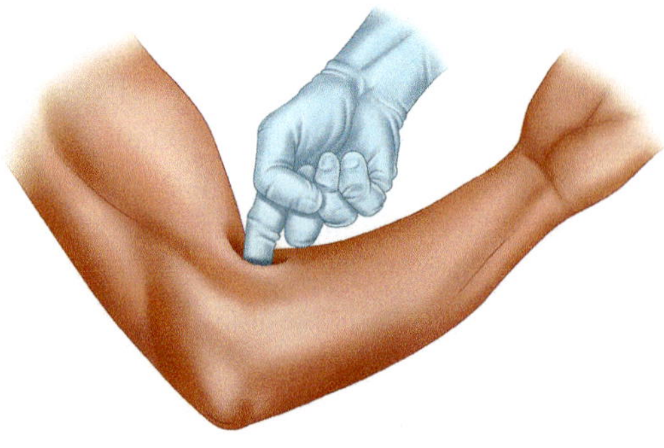

Fig. 8.1 The hook-test

Surgery Related Anatomy

The biceps brachii muscle is composed of two heads: the long head originates from the supraglenoid tubercle, and the short head originates from the coracoid process. Both heads insert distally onto the radial tuberosity. The biceps muscle functions as the primary supinator of the forearm and the secondary flexor of the forearm along with the brachialis. It is inenervated by the musculocutaneous nerve.

There are anatomical variations of the distal biceps tendon. Eames et al. described in a cadavercic study a complete bifurcation of the distal biceps tendon in 10 of 17 specimens [10]. The tendon continued from each muscle belly and inserted distal in two distinct parts. The authors could show that the short head inserts distal to the radial tuberosity and is positioned to be a more powerful flexor of the elbow. The long head inserts further away from the central axis of rotation of the forearm and thereby providing more powerful supination. In an other cadver study, Kulshreshtha et al. analyzed the complex fiber arrangement of the distal biceps tendon [11]. The tendon fibers spiral in a predictable pattern distally to the bicipital aponeurosis, spiraling clockwise in left elbows and counterclockwise in right elbows. Furthermore, the anteromedial fibers follow a relatively straight course and attach inferiorly while the posterolateral fibers coiled beneath the medial fibers to their superior insertion on the tuberosity. The semilunar footprint of the distal biceps insertion is located on the postero-ulnar rim of the tuberosity. There are different types of this postero-ulnar rim which may serve as a pulley to increase the supination strength [12].

The lacertus fibrosus (bicipital aponeurosis), originates from the distal tendon as it passes anterior to the elbow joint and expands ulnarly, blending with the fascia of the forearm and serving as a stabilizer to the distal tendon (Fig. 8.2). As the forearm flexors contract, they tense the lacertus, subsequently causing a medial pull on the biceps tendon and perhaps contributing to its rupture [10, 13]. Only if the lacerus fibrosus is affected, the tendon is completely retracted with a consecutive cranalisation ot the muscle belly.

Therapeutic Options

Conservative Treatment

Conservative treatment should be reserved for older, low-demand patients or those patients with significant medical comorbidities resulting in an unacceptably high risk for surgery. This therapy concept is widely accepted since two studies in the 1980s demnostrated better supination strength as well as flexion strength and endurance after surgical procedure [14, 15]. More recently, Chillemi et al. reported superior clinical outcomes in a small cohort of five patients treated operatively as compared to four patients managed conservatively [16]. Hetsronie et al. also showed similar results in a larger study group of 22 patients [17]. They reported that there was higher subjective satisfaction and higher isokinetic strength and endurance in elbow flexion and forearm supination in the group with surgical reconstruction. In a recent retrospective study, Freeman et al. evaluated 18 patients with an unrepaired dis-

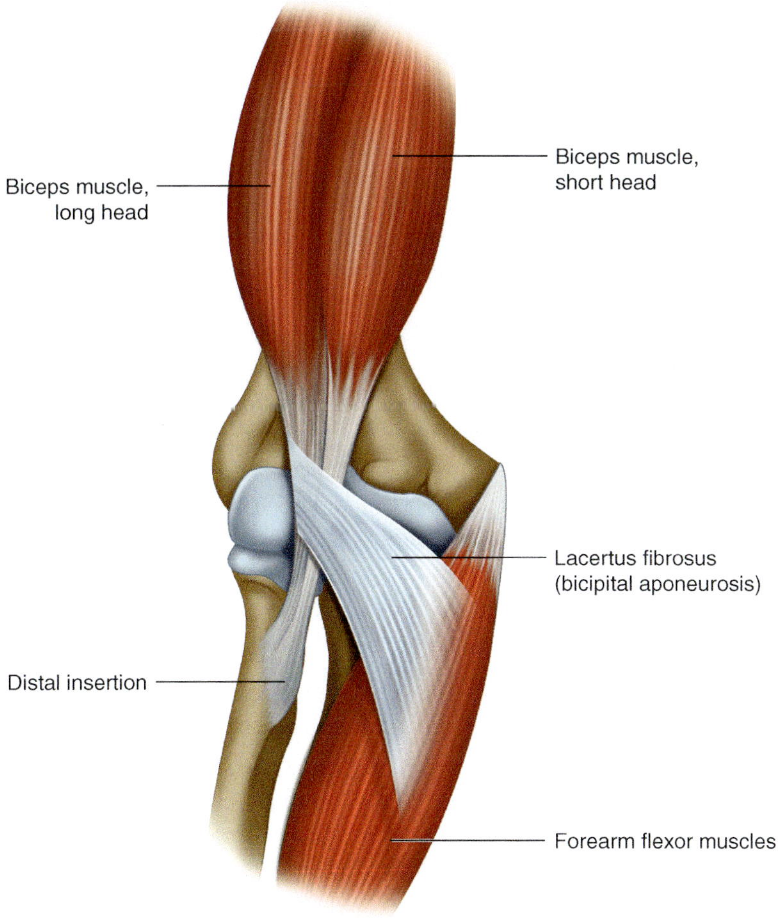

Fig. 8.2 Schematic of distal biceps anatomy (left)

tal biceps tendon rupture and compared them with historical controls who had been treated operatively [18]. There was a significant difference in the supination strength both in comparison to the contralateral side and in comparison to the operated patients. However, the patients treated conservatively achieved good functional results with 95 points in the Mayo Elbow Performance Score (MEPS) and 9 points in the Disability in Arm, Shoulder and Hand score (DASH).

Overall, most studies suggest that better patient outcomes are obtained with surgical treatment. Nonoperative treatment is generally reserved for sedentary patients with low functional requierements or for patients who are not medically fit for operative treatment. The conservative treatment consists of temporary immobilization, pain control, and physiotherapy. Although some chronic activity related pain may occur after nonoperative treatment, satisfactory results can still be expected [18].

Operative Treatment

The operative treatment is the therapy of choice for distal biceps tendon ruptures, as otherwise a loss of supination strength is likely. There are different aspects of the operative treatment. The surgeon has to choose between anatomic or nonanatomic reconstruction, between single-incision or double-incision technique and between several fixation techniques including suture anchors, interference screws, or cortical button based constructs.

When operative treatment became common for distal biceps tendon ruptures, there was discussion about anatomic fixation to the radial tuberosity versus nonanatomic reattachment to the brachialis muscle. With nonanatomic fixation a recovery of supination strength cannot be expected because the tendon is not attached to the lever arm of the tuberosity radii. In a review of 147 cases reported in the literature, Rantanen and Orava noted a 90% rate of good or excellent results at an average of 3 years after anatomic reattachment and a 60% rate of good or excellent results at an average of 3 years following nonanatomic reattachment [19]. Therefore an anatomical reconstruction should always be attempted.

Double-Incision

In its beginning the anatomical reconstruction was achieved by reinserting the tendon transosseosly at the tuberosity radii via a single-incision approach with extensive deep soft tissue preparation. This extensile volar approach (according to Henry – [20]) was associated with a high rate of nerve injuries as reported by Meherin and Kilgore [21]. That's why Boyd and Anderson introduced 1961 the double-incision technique with an additional postero-lateral approach [22]. They noted that the double-incision technique allowed both a lower rate of nerve injury and a more anatomic reattachment of the distal biceps tendon. However this technique involve some stripping of the interosseous membrane with the risk of heterotopic ossification or radioulnar synostosis. To decrease the risk of symptomatic heterotopic ossification, Failla et al. described a modification of the classic Boyd and Anderson approach with limited splitting of the extensor muscles and preservation of the proximal ulnar periosteum [23].

Karunakar et al. performed a retrospective, 4-year follow-up review of 21 patients treated with this modified Boyd-Anderson repair [24]. Almost half of the patients had a deficit in supination strength and 19% of patients demonstrated decreased forearm rotation. The total complication rate was 35% with a 14% incidence of heterotopic ossification and a complete radioulnar synostosis in one patient. Despite these results, they reported good to excellent DASH scores in 20 of 21 patients.

Weinstein et al. performed a retrospective review of 32 patients with distal biceps ruptures treated with the use of suture anchors through the two-incision approach [25]. They did not found any significant differences for strength, endurance and range of motion compared to the uninjured side. The most common complication was transient lateral antebrachial cutaneous nerve palsy. Heterotopic ossifications did not occur.

Single-Incision

Renewed interest in the single-incision approach came with the introduction of modern anchoring systems, which allow a reinsertion via a minimally invasive ventral approach. The theoretical benefit of the single-incision approach is a reduced risk of radioulnar synostosis as the ulnar periosteum is not exposed.

McKee et al. reported the results of 53 patients who had been treated with suture anchor tendon fixation through a single anterior incision [26]. None of the patients lost more than 5° in the flexion-extension or pronation-supination arc. The average DASH score was 8.2 points, which was not substantially different from the average score of 6.2 points in a group of healthy controls. The authors noted four complications: two transient paresthesias of the lateral antebrachial cutaneous nerve, one transient posterior interosseous nerve palsy, and one wound infection. John et al. reported similar results in a retrospective review of 53 patients treated with the single-incision approach using two suture anchors for fixation [27]. They reported all excellent or good Andrews-Carson validated outcomes scores with only a 5.6% complication rate. There were two cases in the series of patients with resultant heterotopic ossification with limited forearm rotation. In one case there was a transient lesion of the N. radialis with consecutive drop hand, which completely recovered in 8 weeks.

Single- Versus Double-Incision

Due to the varied insertion of the distal biceps tendon to the tuberosity radii (as described above), there is the potential risk for a too much anterior tendon fixation when using the single-incision-technique. Hasan et al. evaluated in a cadaveric study the footprint coverage from both the single- and double-incision approaches [28]. The accuracy of a bone tunnel within the original tendon footprint was higher when drilled via a posterolateral approach. Because of rather fixating the tendon in the anterior regions of the tuberosity, the single incision technique might result in a loss of supination torque. However, Henry et al. noted in a biomechanical study that there are no differences in supination or flexion torques between the single- and double-incision technique [29]. This is also reflected in the clinical results. To the best of our knowledge, there is only one prospective, randomized controlled study comparing single- and double-incision technique [30]. Forty-seven patients received a single-incision repair with use of two suture anchors and 44 patients received a double-incision repair with use of transosseous drill holes. After a follow up of 2 years, there were no significant differences in the outcomes between the two groups. Furthermore, there were no differences in isometric extension, pronation, or supination strength at more than 1 year except a minor advantage in final flexion strength with the double-incision technique. Thus for normal daily activities, it seems obvious that a "semi"-anatomic, anterior stump fixation has no effect on functional outcome. In addition, anatomic reinsertion techniques via double-incision are also not able to restore normal supination strength when compared to the uninjured arm [31]. Schmitt et al. supposed a supinator damage during posterior approach as cause for supination weakness due to muscle fat content [32].

Chavan et al. compared in systematic review the clinical outcomes of single-incision and double-incision techniques [33]. Inclusion criteria consisted of an acute repair and at least 1 year of follow-up with the examination including objective strength and motion testing. Unsatisfactory results were significantly more common in the two-incision group (31%) than in the single-incision group (6%), due primarily to decreased forearm rotation or supination strength. Complication rates were similar in the two groups (18% for a single incision and 16% for two incisions); however, the single- incision group had a higher rate of nerve injury (12%) whereas the double- incision group had more frequent loss of forearm rotation (9%). Similarly in the study of Grewal et al., the single incision technique was associated with transient neurapraxias of the lateral antebrachial cutaneous nerve [30]. The differences, however, were marginal so that the authors favored none of both techniques.

Recently, Dunphy et al. analyzed in a retrospective cohort study the complications of 784 distal biceps tendon repairs [34]. When comparing double-incision and single-incision repairs, there was a significantly higher rate of posterior interosseous nerve palsy (3.4% vs 0.8%), heterotopic bone formation (7.6% vs 2.7%), and reoperation (8.3% vs 2.3%) for the double incision technique. The most common complication overall was a lateral antebrachial cutaneous nerve palsy.

To sum up, in the current literature the evidence of superiority of one approach/technique over the other is lacking.

Fixation Methods

The optimal type of fixation of the distal biceps tendon is currently controversially discussed in the literature. For long time the gold standard were bone tunnels. In the meantime, however, numerous new fixation techniques are used. The commonly used methods are suture anchors, cortical buttons and interference screws. Cortical buttons have been found to have the highest load to failure of all techniques [35, 36].

Mazzocca et al. performed a cadaveric biomechanical study comparing the relative strengths of the four most commonly used fixation types; bone tunnels, suture anchors, interference screws and cortical buttons [36]. The cortical button was found to have the significantly higher load to failure than the other three techniques, with no significant difference in displacement rates after cyclical loading.

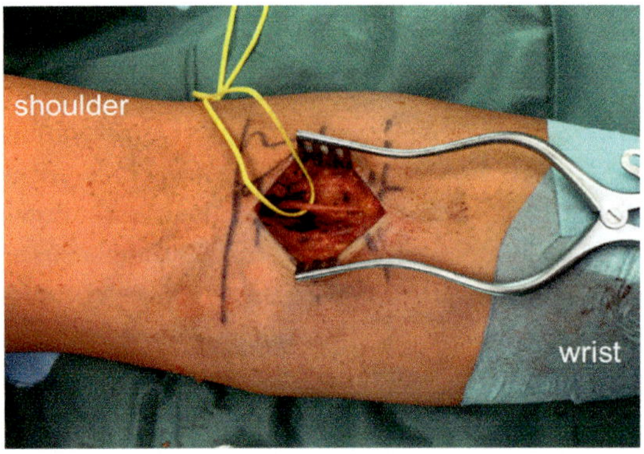

Fig. 8.3 Longitudinal incision distal to antecubital fossa and identification of the LACN (yellow loop)

Given the superior biomechanical properties of cortical button fixation and increased use of this technique, the safety of the posterior interosseous nerve (PIN) was brought into question while drilling through the posterior cortex. PIN injuries have been reported to occur up to 11% of the patients with cortical button repair via single anterior approach [37]. Most of the PIN palsies are transient and resolve during months after surgery; nevertheless, the risk of a permanent nerve injury remains [38].

Author's Preferred Procedure

In order to decrease the risk of injury to the posterior interosseous nerve as a major iatrogenic complication we developed the intramedullary cortical button technique [39]. The intramedullary cortical button positioning enables the repair of the distal biceps tendon to its anatomic footprint without perforating the posterior cortex and consequently not affecting the PIN. After the biomechanical testing has shown very promising results with respect to fixation strength to the bone and displacement, we use this technique in the clinical practice [39, 40]. In the following, the technique is shown in in summarized form:

A longitudinal incision is performed from the distal end of the tuberosity to the antecubital flexion crease (Fig. 8.3). The lateral antebrachial cutaneous nerve is identified, preserved, and retracted laterally. The biceps tendon bursa is opened to expose the retracted tendon stump. Then, the biceps muscle is carefully mobilized with blunt dissection and the radial tuberosity is exposed and roughened for tendon reattachment.

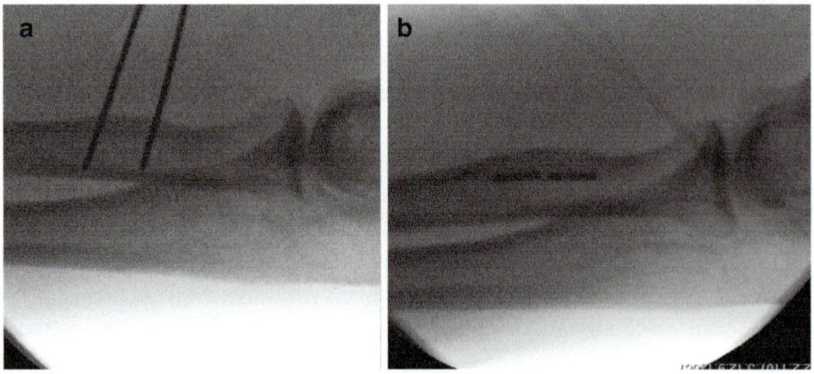

Fig. 8.4 (**a**) Intraoperative control of the positioning of the K-wires, which mark the intended drill holes. In a radius with a smaller diameter, a more flat drilling angle may be required (at least 60°) for smoothly button inserting. (**b**) Intraoperative control of the buttons flipped into the intramedullary canal

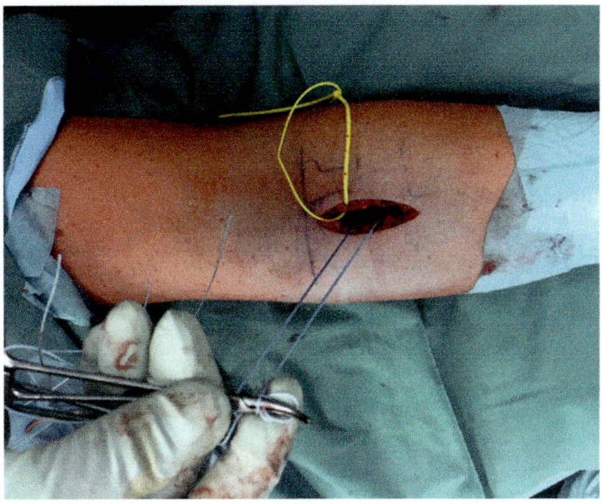

Fig. 8.5 After button flipping each suture has to be strongly tightened, first to test the anchoring of the buttons and second to compress the cancellous bone at the intramedullary canal

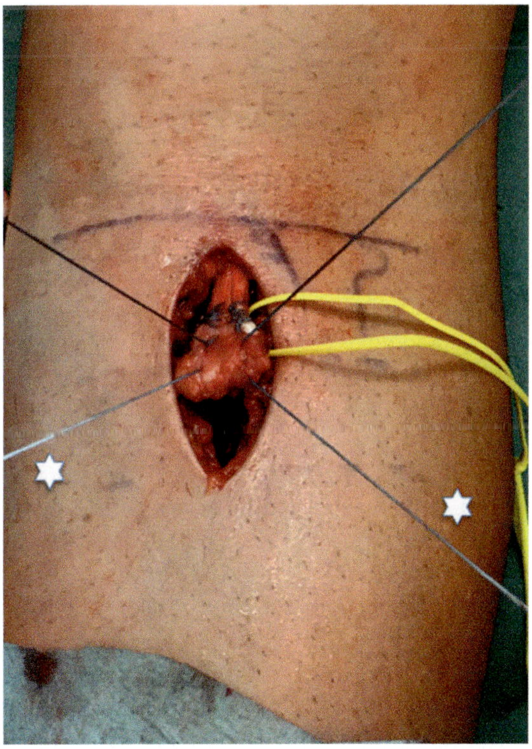

Fig. 8.6 Both free ends (stars) of the FibreWire sutures are simultaneously tightened to deliver the distal biceps tendon to the radial tuberosity

For double intramedullary cortical button implantation, two 2.0 mm K-wires are primary intro-

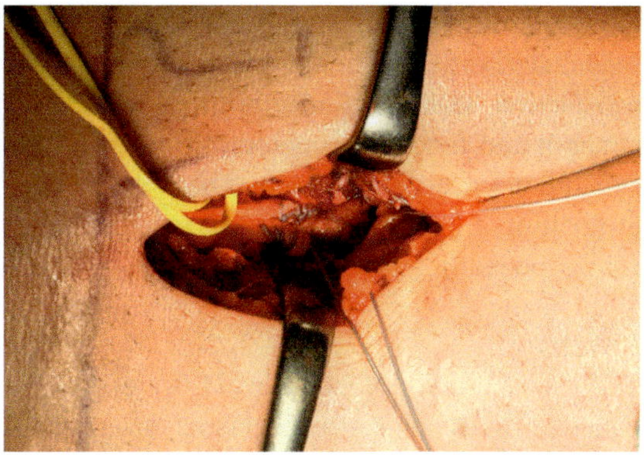

Fig. 8.7 The distal biceps tendon drawn to the radial tuberosity

duced at the radial tuberosity at an angle of 60° to the radial shaft (inclined toward the radial head) to ensure correct positioning of the BicepsButtons ((Arthrex, Naples, FL, USA). To prevent the buttons from interfering with each other inside the medullary canal, a minimum of 12 mm (= length of one BicepsButton) distance between both K-wires has to be observed. The position is controlled by biplanar fluoroscopic imaging (Fig. 8.4a). Next, the 3.2-mm drill holes are performed only into the anterior cortex according to the trajectory of the K-wires. After drilling, the BicepsButtons are passed through the anterior cortex with a Button Inserter (Arthrex, Naples, FL, USA) and flipped. The button position should also be controlled fluoroscopically to rule out insufficient flipping (Fig. 8.4b). Before implanting, both BicepsButtons are single loaded with one nonabsorbable suture (No. 2 FibreWire, Arthrex, Naples, FL, USA). Each suture has to be strongly tightened after button flipping to compress cancellous bone at the intramedullary canal of the radial tuberosity (Fig. 8.5). Then, the distal biceps tendon stump is freshened and sutured using continuous "baseball stitches" with one end of both FibreWires. The other suture end of each FibreWire is used as a lead suture to move the tendon to the radial tuberosity simultaneously (Figs. 8.6 and 8.7). With the elbow in 20° of flexion and full supination, both suture ends are locked directly to the surface of the tuberosity. Skin closure is performed in a standard manner.

The clinical results are promising. The intramedullary cortical button provides high patient's satisfaction and good results with respect to strength and functional outcome. Lesions of the PIN did not occur in any case. The exact clinical evaluation of this technique is subject of a recent follow-up study.

Pitfalls

There are several pitfalls to avoid. Care must be taken to avoid injury to the lateral antebrachial cutaneous nerve. It is usually retracted with the lateral skin flap. Too much pull with the retractors puts the nerve at risk. Venous vessels and the radial recurrent vessels deep in the wound are preserved if possible; otherwise, they are ligated or cauterized enough to get a good visualization of the biceps tuberosity. A good exposition of the biceps tuberosity is required for optimal placement of the drilling holes. Furthermore, the drilling direction is very important to ensure easy button inserting in the intramedullary canal. The drilling into the anterior cortex should be performed at an angle of at least 60° (inclined toward the radial head), especially when the radius has a smaller diameter. Copious irrigation of the situs to remove drilling dust should routinely perform at this point in order to prevent HOs. After button insertion, correct implant anchoring has to be tested clinically and radiologically to prevent secondary button dislocation. The tightening of the tendon to the bone should be done under visualization to avoid soft tissue entrapment and to ensure a firm bone-tendon-contact.

Postoperative Care

In our procedure, immediately after surgery, the patient is stabilized in a posterior splint in 90° elbow flexion. Passive and active (gravity-assisted) motion started under physiotherapist's supervision at 2 days postoperatively. A mobile, hinged brace limiting the last 20° of extension was applied for 4 weeks to secure tendon repair without maximum extension loads. Patients were not allowed active supination, and passive supination, however, was not limited. After 4 weeks, the brace was removed and pain-free active extension and forearm rotation were initiated. Unrestricted activities were commenced at 6 weeks postoperatively; resistance exercises 8 weeks after surgery. Sporting activities were allowed after 12 weeks.

Complications

The most common complication after both single- and double- incision technique is nerve palsy. Particularly, the cutaneous nerve antebrachii (sensitive branch of the musculocutaneous nerve) is endangered. A further complication is the occurrence of heterotopic ossifications at the radial tuberosity. The incidence of heterotopic ossification and radioulnar synostosis appears to be higher with the two-incision approach, although cases of motion limiting heterotopic ossification have been reported after the one-incision approach. Overall, the complication rate varies depending on the study. It can be distinguished between the two approach techniques, but the incidence is not significantly different at all.

Cain et al. reviewed the complication rate in a cohort of 188 patients that underwent the single-incision technique for repair and reported a complication rate of 36% [41]. Minor complications included lateral antebrachial cutaneous nerve paresthesia (26%), radial sensory nerve paresthesia (6%), and superficial infection (2%). Major complications included posterior interosseous nerve injury (4%), symptomatic heterotropic ossification (HO) (3%) and re-rupture (2%). In this series, the use of radiographs was not routine, which may explains the low rate of HOs of just 3%. Other studies report a higher rate of HOs up to 39%, but in most cases they are clinical asymptomatic [42].

Kelly et al. reviewed the complications in a cohort of 78 patients that underwent the double-incision technique for repair and reported a complication rate of 31%. The most common problems were transient nerve palsy (8%, most commonly lateral antebrachial cutaneous nerve) or persistent elbow pain (8%). Asymptomatic HOs were noted in 5%, a superficial wound infection in 4% and a re-rupture in 1%.

Partial Ruptures

Partial ruptures often present in a delayed fashion with persistent pain in the antecubital fossa. Physical examination demonstrates a painful limited supination and flexion strength with a still palpable distal biceps tendon. MRI is capable of quantifying the extent of the tear, as well as differentiating other relevant diseases. Partial ruptures involving greater than 50% of the insertion should be taken down during surgery and treated as a complete rupture with reattachment using standard techniques [43].

Recently Behun et al. reviewed the literature regarding surgical outcomes for treatment of partial tears of the distal biceps brachii tendon with varied surgical approaches and fixation [44]. The review involved 19 studies with 85 patients. Surgery resulted in 94% satisfactory clinical outcome which meant less than 30° range of motion loss in all directions, supination and flexion strength greater than 80% compared with the contralateral extremity, and absence of major complication such as surgical revision or persistent nerve injury. Complication rates were similar to other series of acute repairs.

Analogous to the technique introduced by Kelly et al. [45], partial distal biceps tendon ruptures can be treated with the aforementioned intramedullary button technique through a single posterior incision. The morbidity of the anterior exposure can be avoided and the exact anatomical tendon footprint readily explored. The remaining tendon is released and reattached with the intramedullary button technique at its original footprint [31].

Chronic Ruptures

In cases of chronic distal biceps ruptures, the combination of muscle atrophy, distal tendon retraction, and fibrosis makes primary anatomic reattachment of the tendon particularly challenging. The choice of therapy must be made dependent on the functional demand and the general condition of the patient. In the case of a low functional demand, a conservative procedure or an extraanatomic fixation (insertion of the distal biceps tendon on the musculotendinous transition of the lower muscle layer of brachialis and brachioradialis as a low-risk method for improving the loss of strength) should be indicated [46]. For patients with high physical demands, the reconstruction of the distal biceps tendon with a tendon graft is recommended [47]. Augmentation options include fascia lata, M. flexor carpi radialis or semitendinosus and Achilles tendon.

Wiley et al. compared the results of 7 patients who underwent reconstruction of a chronic rupture with a semitendinosus allograft and seven patients who were treated nonoperatively [48]. In the surgical group flexion and supination strength was restored to the normal range whereas the nonoperative had a residual 20% strength deficit. The Endurance in both groups was within the normal range.

There are several retrospective studies in the literature evaluating the results of chronic distal biceps rupture reconstructions. All have relatively low numbers of patients with varied graft choices. Overall, excellent results were noted after the reconstructions with restoration of strength and endurance in most cases [49–51].

References

1. Kelly MP, et al. Distal biceps tendon ruptures: an epidemiological analysis using a large population database. Am J Sports Med. 2015;43(8):2012–7.
2. Safran MR, Graham SM. Distal biceps tendon ruptures: incidence, demographics, and the effect of smoking. Clin Orthop Relat Res. 2002;404:275–83
3. Pagonis T, et al. The effect of steroid-abuse on anatomic reinsertion of ruptured distal biceps brachii tendon. Injury. 2011;42(11):1307–12.
4. D'Alessandro DF, et al. Repair of distal biceps tendon ruptures in athletes. Am J Sports Med. 1993;21(1):114–9.
5. Seiler JG 3rd, et al. The distal biceps tendon. Two potential mechanisms involved in its rupture: arterial supply and mechanical impingement. J Shoulder Elbow Surg. 1995;4(3):149–56.
6. Ruland RT, Dunbar RP, Bowen JD. The biceps squeeze test for diagnosis of distal biceps tendon ruptures. Clin Orthop Relat Res. 2005;437:128–31.
7. O'Driscoll SW, Goncalves LB, Dietz P. The hook test for distal biceps tendon avulsion. Am J Sports Med. 2007;35(11):1865–9.
8. Belli P, et al. Sonographic diagnosis of distal biceps tendon rupture: a prospective study of 25 cases. J Ultrasound Med. 2001;20(6):587–95.

9. Giuffre BM, Moss MJ. Optimal positioning for MRI of the distal biceps brachii tendon: flexed abducted supinated view. AJR Am J Roentgenol. 2004;182(4):944–6.
10. Eames MH, et al. Distal biceps tendon anatomy: a cadaveric study. J Bone Joint Surg Am. 2007;89(5):1044–9.
11. Kulshreshtha R, et al. Anatomy of the distal biceps brachii tendon and its clinical relevance. Clin Orthop Relat Res. 2007;456:117–20.
12. Mazzocca AD, et al. The anatomy of the bicipital tuberosity and distal biceps tendon. J Shoulder Elb Surg. 2007;16(1):122–7.
13. Athwal GS, Steinmann SP, Rispoli DM. The distal biceps tendon: footprint and relevant clinical anatomy. J Hand Surg Am. 2007;32(8):1225–9.
14. Baker BE, Bierwagen D. Rupture of the distal tendon of the biceps brachii. Operative versus non-operative treatment. J Bone Joint Surg Am. 1985;67(3):414–7.
15. Morrey BF, et al. Rupture of the distal tendon of the biceps brachii. A biomechanical study. J Bone Joint Surg Am. 1985;67(3):418–21.
16. Chillemi C, Marinelli M, De Cupis V. Rupture of the distal biceps brachii tendon: conservative treatment versus anatomic reinsertion–clinical and radiological evaluation after 2 years. Arch Orthop Trauma Surg. 2007;127(8):705–8.
17. Hetsroni I, et al. Avulsion of the distal biceps brachii tendon in middle-aged population: is surgical repair advisable? A comparative study of 22 patients treated with either nonoperative management or early anatomical repair. Injury. 2008;39(7):753–60.
18. Freeman CR, et al. Nonoperative treatment of distal biceps tendon ruptures compared with a historical control group. J Bone Joint Surg Am. 2009;91(10):2329–34.
19. Rantanen J, Orava S. Rupture of the distal biceps tendon. A report of 19 patients treated with anatomic reinsertion, and a meta-analysis of 147 cases found in the literature. Am J Sports Med. 1999;27(2):128–32.
20. Henry AK. Extensile exposures. Edinburgh: Churchill Livingston; 1973. p. 19.
21. Meherin JM, Kilgore ES. The treatment of ruptures of the distal biceps brachii tendon. Am J Surg. 1960;99:636–40.
22. Boyd HB, Anderson LD. A method for reinsertion of the distal biceps brachii tendon. J Bone Joint Surg Am. 1961;43:1041–3.
23. Failla JM, et al. Proximal radioulnar synostosis after repair of distal biceps brachii rupture by the two-incision technique. Report of four cases. Clin Orthop Relat Res. 1990;253:133–6.
24. Karunakar MA, Cha P, Stern PJ. Distal biceps ruptures. A followup of Boyd and Anderson repair. Clin Orthop Relat Res. 1999;363:100–7.
25. Weinstein DM, et al. Elbow function after repair of the distal biceps brachii tendon with a two-incision approach. J Shoulder Elbow Surg. 2008;17(1 Suppl):82S–6S.
26. McKee MD, et al. Patient-oriented functional outcome after repair of distal biceps tendon ruptures using a single-incision technique. J Shoulder Elbow Surg. 2005;14(3):302–6.
27. John CK, et al. Single-incision repair of acute distal biceps ruptures by use of suture anchors. J Shoulder Elbow Surg. 2007;16(1):78–83.
28. Hasan SA, et al. Two-incision versus one-incision repair for distal biceps tendon rupture: a cadaveric study. J Shoulder Elbow Surg. 2012;21(7):935–41.
29. Henry J, et al. Biomechanical analysis of distal biceps tendon repair methods. Am J Sports Med. 2007;35(11):1950–4.
30. Grewal R, et al. Single versus double-incision technique for the repair of acute distal biceps tendon ruptures: a randomized clinical trial. J Bone Joint Surg Am. 2012;94(13):1166–74.
31. Schmidt CC, Savoie FH 3rd, Steinmann SP, et al. Distal biceps tendon history, updates, and controversies: from the closed American shoulder and elbow surgeons meeting-2015. J Shoulder Elbow Surg. 2016;25(10):1717–30.
32. Schmidt CC, Brown BT, Qvick LM, et al. Factors that determine supination strength following distal biceps repair. J Bone Joint Surg Am. 2016;98(14):1153–60.
33. Chavan PR, Duquin TR, Bisson LJ. Repair of the ruptured distal biceps tendon: a systematic review. Am J Sports Med. 2008;36(8):1618–24.
34. Dunphy TR, et al. Surgical treatment of distal biceps tendon ruptures: an analysis of complications in 784 surgical repairs. Am J Sports Med. 2017;45(13):3020–9.
35. Kettler M, et al. Failure strengths in distal biceps tendon repair. Am J Sports Med. 2007;35(9):1544–8.
36. Mazzocca AD, et al. Biomechanical evaluation of 4 techniques of distal biceps brachii tendon repair. Am J Sports Med. 2007;35(2):252–8.
37. Banerjee M, et al. High complication rate following distal biceps refixation with cortical button. Arch Orthop Trauma Surg. 2013;133(10):1361–6.
38. Van den Bogaerde J, Shin E. Posterior interosseous nerve incarceration with endobutton repair of distal biceps. Orthopedics. 2015;38(1):e68–71.
39. Siebenlist S, et al. Biomechanical in vitro validation of intramedullary cortical button fixation for distal biceps tendon repair: a new technique. Am J Sports Med. 2011;39(8):1762–8.
40. Siebenlist S, et al. Double intramedullary cortical button versus suture anchors for distal biceps tendon repair: a biomechanical comparison. Knee Surg Sports Traumatol Arthrosc. 2015;23(3):926–33.
41. Cain RA, et al. Complications following distal biceps repair. J Hand Surg Am. 2012;37(10):2112–7.
42. Siebenlist S, et al. The functional outcome of forty-nine single-incision suture anchor repairs for distal biceps tendon ruptures at the elbow. Int Orthop. 2014;38(4):873–9.
43. Bain GI, Johnson LJ, Turner PC. Treatment of partial distal biceps tendon tears. Sports Med Arthrosc. 2008;16(3):154–61.

44. Behun MA, et al. Partial tears of the distal biceps brachii tendon: a systematic review of surgical outcomes. J Hand Surg Am. 2016;41(7):e175–89.
45. Kelly EW, Steinmann S, O'Driscoll SW. Surgical treatment of partial distal biceps tendon ruptures through a single posterior incision. J Shoulder Elbow Surg. 2003;12(5):456–61.
46. Darlis NA, Sotereanos DG. Distal biceps tendon reconstruction in chronic ruptures. J Shoulder Elbow Surg. 2006;15(5):614–9.
47. Snir N, et al. Clinical outcomes after chronic distal biceps reconstruction with allografts. Am J Sports Med. 2013;41(10):2288–95.
48. Wiley WB, et al. Late reconstruction of chronic distal biceps tendon ruptures with a semitendinosus autograft technique. J Shoulder Elbow Surg. 2006;15(4):440–4.
49. Vastamaki M, Vastamaki H. A simple grafting method to repair irreparable distal biceps tendon. Clin Orthop Relat Res. 2008;466(10):2475–81.
50. Levy HJ, Mashoof AA, Morgan D. Repair of chronic ruptures of the distal biceps tendon using flexor carpi radialis tendon graft. Am J Sports Med. 2000;28(4):538–40.
51. Sanchez-Sotelo J, et al. Reconstruction of chronic ruptures of the distal biceps tendon with use of an achilles tendon allograft. J Bone Joint Surg Am. 2002;84-A(6):999–1005.

9

Total Elbow Arthroplasty in the Treatment of Complex Distal Humeral Fractures

Jeremy Alan Hall

Introduction

Total elbow arthroplasty has been a reliable method of treatment for elbow arthritis for over 40 years [1–5]. The indications for total elbow arthroplasty have continued to expand to include the management of acute traumatic and post-traumatic conditions. Cobb and Morrey proposed the use of non-custom total elbow replacement for the treatment of complex distal humeral fractures in the elderly in 1997 [6]. The role of total elbow arthroplasty for the management of complex distal humeral fractures has met much debate since.

Distal humeral fractures frequently occur in patients over the age of 60 years, often as a result of low energy injuries such as a fall from standing height. In osteoporotic bone, these low energy injuries often produce complex intra-articular fractures and comminution that can challenge the Orthopaedic surgeon. Furthermore, individuals in this age group often suffer from significant medical comorbidities, and frequently require increased upper extremity assistance in typical activities of daily living, such as in use of mobility aides, and for assistance rising from the seated position. This can lead to challenges in the post-operative period, and occasionally, "non-compliance" with typical post-operative use and weight bearing recommendations, which can lead to fixation failure.

Primary Total Elbow Arthroplasty for Distal Humeral Fractures

Multiple studies have evaluated the effectiveness of total elbow arthroplasty in the treatment of complex intra-articular distal humeral fractures. Early studies in select populations comparing fracture fixation with plate and screw constructs and total elbow arthroplasty found favor in arthroplasty in selected patients.

Frankle et al. (2003) compared 24 women over the age of 65 with complex distal humeral fractures treated with open reduction and internal fixation (ORIF) using standard small fragment fixation and semi-constrained total elbow arthroplasty (TEA) over 57 months. They found the total elbow arthroplasty group to have shorter operative times (146 min ORIF vs 78 min TEA), shorter hospital length of stay (3 days ORIF vs 2 days TEA), improved elbow arc of flexion-extension (100° ORIF vs 113° TEA), and improved functional outcomes (MEPs 81 ORIF vs 95 TEA). In 25% of patients in the ORIF group, fixation failed, requiring revision to total elbow arthroplasty during the follow-up period. At the conclusion of the

J. A. Hall (✉)
University of Toronto, Toronto, ON, Canada
e-mail: hallj@smh.ca

P. Biberthaler et al. (eds.), *Acute Elbow Trauma*, Strategies in Fracture Treatments,
https://doi.org/10.1007/978-3-319-97850-5_9

study, the authors recommended fixation as first line treatment of complex fractures of the distal humerus in women 65 years and older without medical comorbidities and adequate bone stock. However, in those with medical comorbidities, complex fracture patterns, and those with poor bone stock, TEA was a valuable option for treatment [7].

Subsequently, McKee et al. (2009) compared open reduction and internal fixation with total elbow arthroplasty for displaced comminuted intra-articular fractures of the distal humerus with semi-constrained total elbow arthroplasty in male and female patients over the age of 65 years (mean age of 77 years). After 2 years follow up, the authors reported improved functional outcome (DASH and MEPS) in the total elbow group, with a 25% conversion from the ORIF group to the TEA group intra-operatively due to inability to achieve stable fixation [8].

Open injuries offer even greater challenges in the treatment of distal humeral fractures. Linn et al. (2014) reviewed seven patients, mean age 74, with grade 1 and grade 2 open distal humeral fractures after a staged protocol of serial irrigation and debridement, followed by primary total elbow arthroplasty. They describe no wound complications or deep infections using this protocol and suggested that total elbow arthroplasty is a viable treatment option for complex open distal humeral fractures [9].

A systematic review and meta-analysis by Githens et al. in 2014 comparing open reduction and internal fixation versus total elbow arthroplasty for the treatment of geriatric distal humeral fractures found similar functional outcomes and range of motion, with a trend toward higher incidence of major complications and reoperation after fixation [10].

Total Elbow Arthroplasty After Failed Fixation

In the setting of failed fracture fixation, total elbow arthroplasty provides a functional range of motion with a complication rate similar to that of primary total elbow arthroplasty for fracture. Prasad and Dent (2008) evaluated 32 patients, 15 in the early total elbow arthroplasty group and 17 in the delayed arthroplasty treatment group, after conservative treatment or failed fixation. After a mean follow-up of over 56 months, there was no significant difference in Mayo performance elbow score or survivorship between the groups, with similar incidence of loosening. The delayed group experienced two deep infections and two patients with ulnar nerve palsy. Despite these complications, no significant differences were found between the groups [11]. As such, complex distal humeral fractures managed with fixation which subsequently fails, revision through arthroplasty replacement can provide acceptable results.

Long Term Outcome of Total Elbow Arthroplasty for Fracture

In the short term, total elbow arthroplasty for fracture yields reasonable function and may provide ongoing independence for frail elderly. However, long term studies suggest poor 10 year survival rates particularly in patients with rheumatoid arthritis. Barco et al. (2017) reported on the 10 year outcomes of 44 patients after total elbow arthroplasty for fracture. Implant revision or resection was performed in 8 elbows for infection (3 elbows), ulnar component loosening (3 elbows), and ulnar component fracture (2 elbows). Periprosthetic fractures were noted in 5 elbows. Survival rates in patients with rheumatoid arthritis were 85% at 5 years and 76% at 10 years, while those without rheumatoid arthritis enjoyed survival rates of 92% at 5 and 10 years. The most relevant risk factor for revision was male sex (hazard ratio 12.6) [12].

These studies provide encouraging insight into the management of these complex injuries, however it should be emphasized that total elbow arthroplasty should be reserved for individuals that can abide by the post-arthroplasty medically imposed restrictions. Elbow arthroplasty does not allow for repetitive or heavy lifting, nor is it recommended to return to such activities as golf or tennis as these activities will inevitably lead to increased wear and early loosening or failure. However, it is generally agreed that fractures in selected elbows with pre-existing arthritis, low demand individuals, and fractures with unreconstructable joint surface injuries could benefit from total elbow arthroplasty. Similarly, for best results and lowest complication rate, total elbow arthroplasty should be undertaken by surgeons experienced in total elbow arthroplasty.

Technique: Total Elbow Arthroplasty for Complex Distal Humeral Fractures - Authors Preferred Method [13]

In the setting of distal humeral fracture, total elbow arthroplasty is typically performed with a semi-constrained or "sloppy hinge" prosthesis.

In the appropriate patient (Fig. 9.1), after regional and/or general anesthetic, the patient is placed in the lateral decubitus position with the affected limb on a bolster (Fig. 9.2). Should the patient's condition not be amenable to the lateral decubitus position, in the supine position, the injured extremity may be supported by rolls or bolsters on the patient's chest or a positioning aid. A tourniquet is applied. Should the fracture extend proximally into the metadiaphysis or diaphysis, and more proximal stabilization is anticipated, a sterile tourniquet may be used.

The arm is carefully prepped and draped to facilitate access to the elbow joint. A posterior surgical approach facilitates access to the triceps fascia. The ulnar nerve is identified and mobilized to facilitate safe access to the elbow joint and fracture. In the setting of total elbow arthroplasty for distal humeral fracture, the author pre-

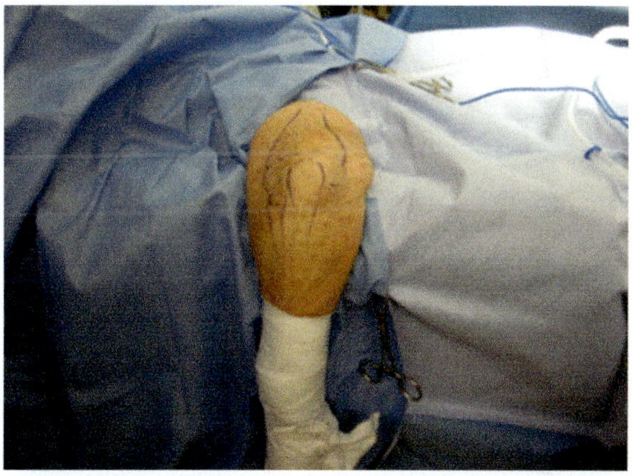

Fig. 9.2 The patient is placed in the lateral decubitus position, with tourniquet applied and the operative arm supported by bolster

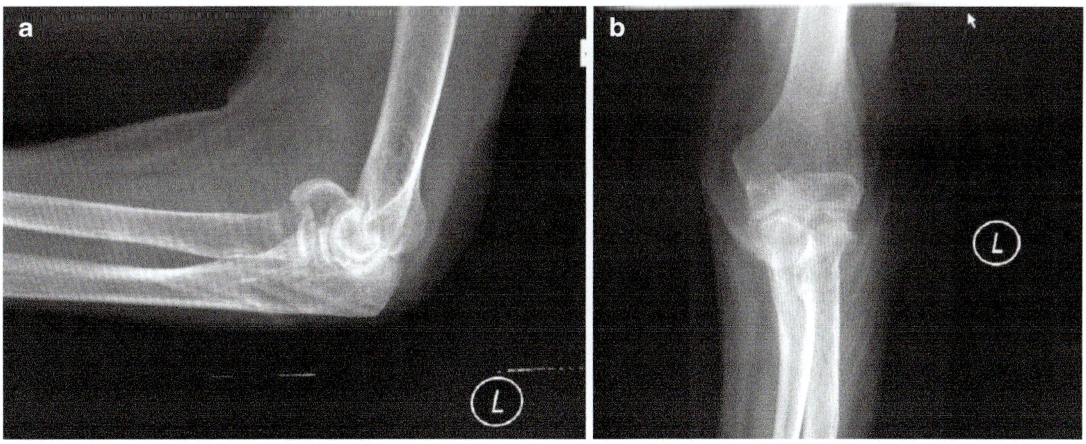

Fig. 9.1 Lateral (**a**) and anteroposterior radiographs (**b**) of an intra-articular fracture of the distal humerus in a 76 year old male

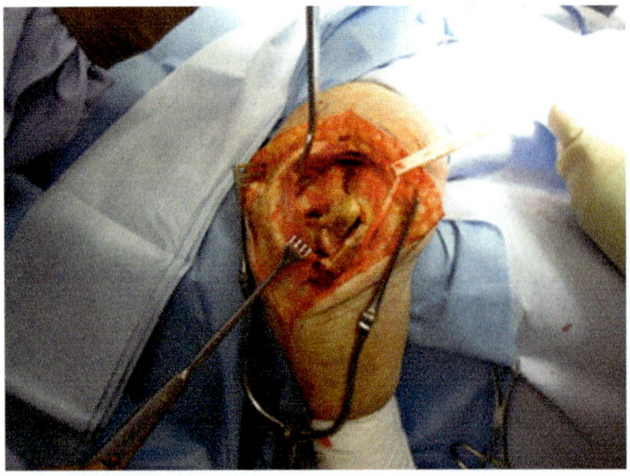

Fig. 9.3 A posterior approach to the elbow utilizing a triceps sparring dissection facilitates adequate visualization of the distal humeral fracture fragments and elbow joint, while facilitating unrestricted elbow motion after surgery. The ulnar nerve is mobilized and protected during the procedure

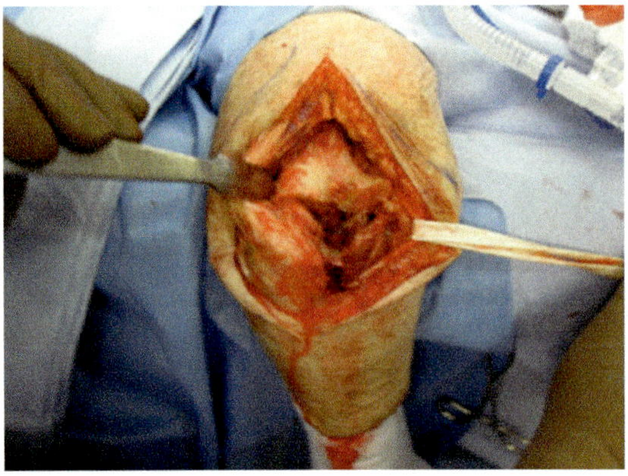

Fig. 9.4 Resection of the distal humeral fracture fragments provides a "working space" to prepare the humerus and ulna for implant

fers a para-tricipital triceps sparing approach (Fig. 9.3). This facilitates early elbow range of motion, strengthening, and upper extremity weight-bearing through an intact triceps attachment. From the medial and lateral para-tricipital portals, the fracture fragments of the distal humerus are skeletonized and removed. This creates a "working space" wherein the humeral shaft and proximal ulna may be accessed and prepared for insertion of the semi-constrained elbow prosthesis (Fig. 9.4).

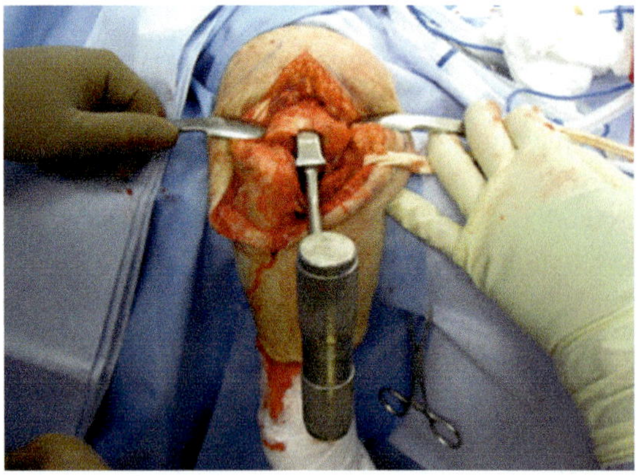

Fig. 9.5 After fracture resection, the distal humerus is prepared with canal reaming and broaching

The humerus is first prepared. With the condyles removed, there is no need to prepare the distal aspect of the humerus. The shaft is progressively reamed and broached to facilitate insertion of the humeral stem (Fig. 9.5). The semiconstrained nature of the prosthesis does not require intact medial or lateral ligaments nor reconstruction, thus allowing condylar resection. If possible, as in total elbow arthroplasty for arthritis, a wedge of bone should be fashioned and placed between the anterior flange of the humeral component and the intact humeral shaft to increase anterior bone density. The height of the prosthesis can be estimated through assembly of the fracture fragments or by soft tissue tensioning at trialing.

The proximal ulna is prepared in standard fashion. The author prefers to remove the tip of the olecranon and create a groove in the articular surface of the ulna with a burr such that the ulnar component could be inserted without impingement. A burr is first used to open the ulnar canal which is followed by progressive rasps (Fig. 9.6). The ulnar component is trialed for fit.

The trial prostheses are then inserted and the elbow reduced and linked (Fig. 9.7). This should facilitate an easy range of motion from approximately 5° of extension to full flexion. As in arthroplasty for arthritis, allowing soft tissue tension to slightly limit elbow extension will prevent

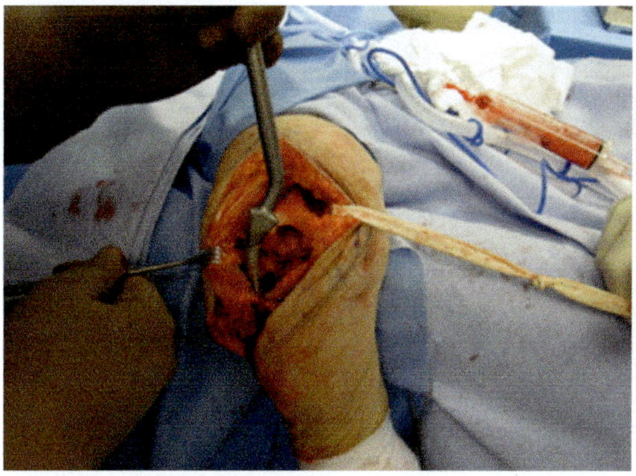

Fig. 9.6 The ulna is prepared in typical fashion, using a burr to identify and prepare the ulnar canal, followed by reaming and broaching

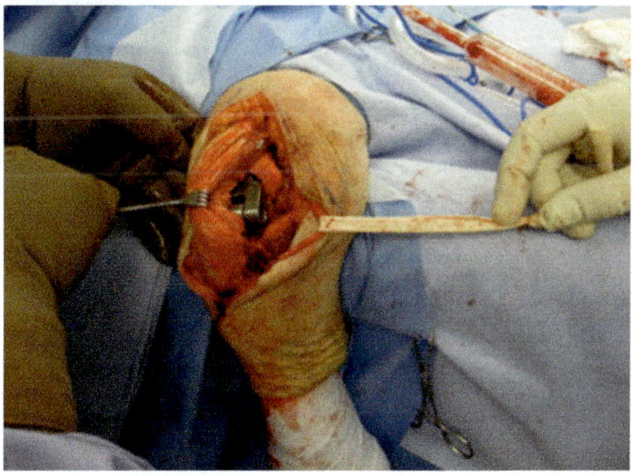

Fig. 9.7 With the trials are introduced, elbow range of motion and soft tissue tension are assessed. The height of the humeral component should be noted. This offers an opportunity to practice implant introduction before cementing

hyperextension of the elbow joint, which could lead to elbow locking. Pronation and supination is typically normal in the fractured elbow, however should there be deficiencies as a result of proximal radial-ulnar disorders or arthritis, the radial head may be excised. A few practice runs in the insertion of the components will allow for a seamless introduction of the components during cementing.

With adequate motion, the position of the humeral component relative to the intact portion

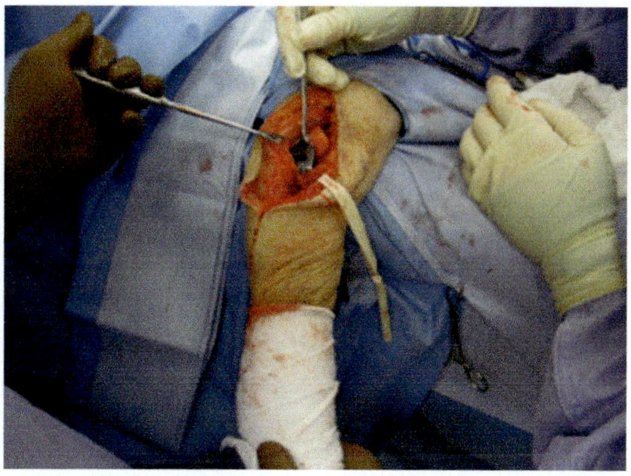

Fig. 9.8 The permanent implants are cemented into place as the trials dictated and the elbow is held in near full extension as the cement cures

of the humeral shaft is noted. Should a significant portion of the humeral shaft be involved in the fracture, consideration should be made for longer stem length humerus.

After selection of the appropriate implants, the permanent humeral and ulnar components are inserted in the same fashion as the trials and are cemented into position. The elbow is reduced and the components are linked. Typically to ensure the components remain well-seated, the elbow is extended to approximate 5° of flexion while the cement cures (Fig. 9.8). Extraneous cement is carefully removed. The anterior aspect of the elbow joint is inspected for residual cement which is removed.

The wound is then copiously irrigated with saline. The medial and lateral para-tricipital apertures are re-approximated with interrupted sutures. The ulnar nerve is left in its natural setting however with condyles removed may tend to sublux anteriorly. Should this be the case, the surgeon may consider anterior transposition to maintain the position of the nerve. The final position of the ulnar nerve is well documented postoperatively.

Postoperatively the wound is dressed and the arm is placed in a plaster splint in a semi-extended position overnight. The splint is removed on the first postoperative day and gentle range of motion exercises may begin (Fig. 9.9).

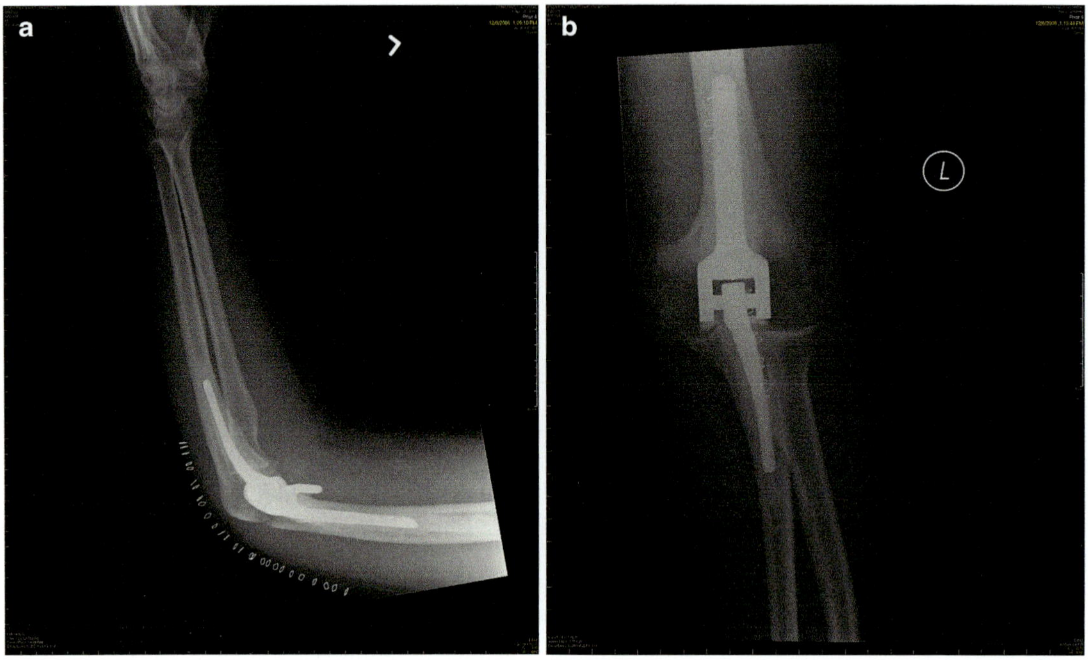

Fig. 9.9 Post-operative lateral (**a**) and anteroposterior (**b**) radiographs of patient in Fig. 9.1

Conclusion

Total elbow arthroplasty in the management of complex intra-articular distal humeral fractures offers advantages in select patient populations. Fractures undergoing fixation frequently take months to achieve sufficient union to provide weight-bearing for activities such as arising from a seated position, upper extremity assisted ambulation, and self-care, in the frail elderly. Total elbow arthroplasty offers immediate stability and thereby allow for immediate active elbow extension and weight-bearing. This could potentially mean the difference between independent and supportive lifestyles for these patients.

Long-term outcome after total elbow arthroplasty for fracture suggests reasonable survivorship at 5 and 10 years post-surgery. In this relatively sedentary and low demand subset of distal humeral fracture, this procedure frequently does not come to revision.

Complex intra-articular distal humeral fracture should be approached with a plan of operative fixation with modern pre-contoured locking plates and technique. Should this not be possible because of bone stock, excessive intra-articular comminution, or pre-existing arthritic disease, consideration could be made for total elbow arthroplasty.

References

1. Aldridge JM III, Light NR, Mallon WJ, Coonrad RW. Total elbow arthroplasty with the Coonrad-Morrey prosthesis: a 10 to 31 year survival analysis. J Bone Joint Surg (Br). 2006;88:509–14.
2. Gill DR, Morrey BF. The Coonrad-Morrey total elbow arthroplasty in patients who have rheumatoid arthritis. A ten to fifteen-year follow-up study. J Bone Joint Surg AM. 1998;80:1327–35.
3. Morrey BF, Adams RA. Semiconstrained arthroplasty for the treatment of rheumatoid arthritis. J Bone Joint Surg Am. 1992;74:479–90.
4. Plasche HC, Thillemann TM, Brorson S, Olsen BS. Implant survival after total elbow arthroplasty: a retrospective study of 324 procedures performed from 1980 to 2008. J Shoulder Elb Surg. 2014;23:829–36.
5. Welsink CL, Lambers KTA, van Deurzen DFP, Eygendaal D, van den Bekerom MPJ. Total elbow arthroplasty: a systematic review. J Bone Joint Surg Reviews. 2017;5(7):e4.

6. Cobb TK, Morrey BF. Total elbow arthroplasty as primary treatment for distal humeral fractures in elderly patients. J Bone Joint Surg Am. 1997;79(6):826–32.
7. Frankle MA, Herscovici D Jr, Dipasquale TG, Vasey MB, Sanders RW. A comparison of open reduction and internal fixation and primary total elbow arthroplasty in the treatment of intraarticular distal humeral fractures in women older than age 65. J Orthop Trauma. 2003;17:473–80.
8. McKee MD, Veillette CJ, Hall JA, Schemitsch EH, Wild LM, McCormack R, Perey B, Goetz T, Zomar M, Moon K, Mandel S, Petit S, Guy P, Leung I. A multicenter, prospective, randomized, controlled trial of open reduction-internal fixation versus total elbow arthroplasty for displaced intra-articular distal humeral fractures in elderly patients. J Shoulder Elb Surg. 2009;18:3–12.
9. Linn MS, Gardner MJ, McAndrew CM, Gallagher B, Ricci WM. Is primary total elbow arthroplasty safe for the treatment of open intra-articular distal humerus fractures? Injury. 2014;45(11):1747–51.
10. Githens M, Yao J, Sox AH, Bishop J. Open reduction and internal fixation versus total elbow arthroplasty for the treatment of geriatric distal humerus fractures: a systematic review and meta-analysis. J Orthop Trauma. 2014;28(8):481–8.
11. Prasad N, Dent C. Outcome of total elbow replacement for distal humerus fractures in the elderly: a comparison of primary surgery and surgery after failed internal fixation or conservative treatment. J Bone Joint Surg Br. 2008;90(3):343–8.
12. Barco R, Streubel PN, Morrey BF, Sanchez-Sotelo J. Total elbow arthroplasty for distal humeral fractures: a ten-year-minimum follow-up study. J Bone Joint Surg. 2017;99(18):1524–31.
13. Hall JA, McKee MD. Total elbow arthroplasty for intra-articular fractures of the distal humerus. Tech Orthop. 2000;15:120–7.

Varia: Vascular Injury

10

Heiko Wendorff, Benedikt Reutersberg, and Hans-Henning Eckstein

Epidemiology

Vascular injuries in upper extremities resulting from acute elbow trauma are very infrequent. The literature only describes case reports or case series. The quantity of arterial ruptures following closed elbow dislocations is quoted by 0.3–1.7% [1, 2]. Only one retrospective study describes general arterial injuries in 13% of the elbow traumas [3].

Because of the anatomical proximity to the neurovascular trunc, a pronounced elbow injury can harm the vessels in this region. In addition to a complete transsection of the vessel the elbow trauma can cause arterial dissections, intimal tears, thrombosis or aneurysms.

Based on the strong collateral system in the upper extremity the peripheral pulse can be palpable even if the artery is completely transsected [3]. The combination of elbow trauma and vascular injury indicates an acute vascular diagnostic and therapy.

Classification

Different kinds of classifications for vascular injuries of the upper extremites were published. The oldest and most common classification (Fig. 10.1) was published 1965 by Lindner and Vollmar, who created a classification system which distinguish between sharp and blunt vascular injuries.

The classification is grouped in three severity grades:

Grade	Explanation
I	Partial transection of the vascular wall, without opening the lumina
II	Vessel opening with partial transection of the vessel
III	Complete transection of the vessel

Another classification system, described by Feliciano et al. in 2009 distinguishes between different types of vascular injuries depending on the underlying pathomechanism [4]. There are five types:

Type	Explanation
I	Intimal injury (flaps, disruptions or subintimal/intramural hematomas)
II	Complete wall defects (Pseudoaneurysm/hemorrhage)
III	Complete transection (hemorrhage, occlusion)
IV	Arteriovenous fistulas
V	Vessel spasm

H. Wendorff (✉) · B. Reutersberg · H.-H. Eckstein
Department of Vascular and Endovascular Surgery, Klinikum rechts der Isar, Technical University of Munich, Munich, Germany
e-mail: heiko.wendorff@mri.tum.de

P. Biberthaler et al. (eds.), *Acute Elbow Trauma*, Strategies in Fracture Treatments,
https://doi.org/10.1007/978-3-319-97850-5_10

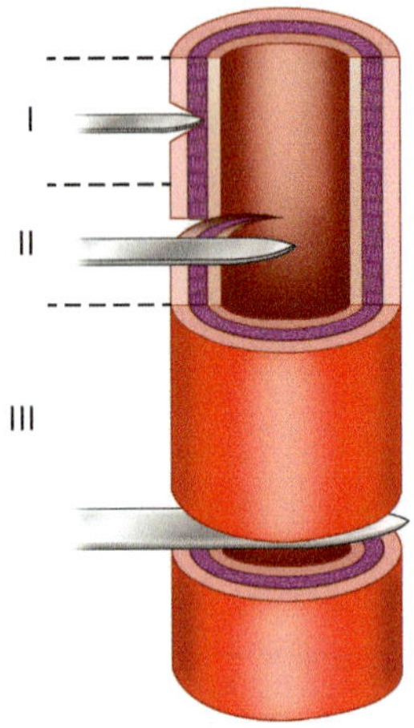

	External bleeding	Peripheral Ischemia
I	ø	ø
II	+++	ø (+)
III	++	+++

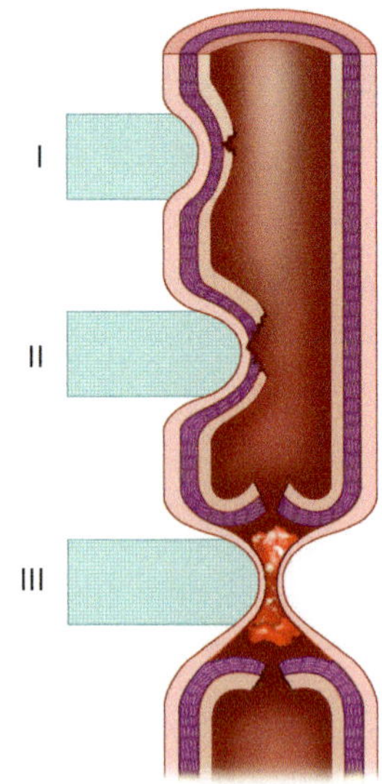

	External bleeding	Peripheral Ischemia
I	ø	ø
II	ø	(+)
III	ø or +	+++

Fig. 10.1 Schematical description of vascular injuries as a function of the injury pattern, including the associated symptoms (by Linder and Vollmar 1965) (Debus, Gross-Fengels Springer (ISBN 978–3–642-01708-7))

Symptoms and Diagnostics

In addition to the test of the motor function during physical examination it is important to evaluate the neurological status and circulation of the extremity [5]. In 2011 Feliciano et al. published an algorithm (Fig. 10.2) for the assessment of patients with suspected peripheral vascular injury [6].

A "Redflag" sign (Hard sign) (Fig. 10.2) for an arterial injury is an external bleeding, a rapid expanding hematoma or any classical sign of arterial occlusion (6 "P"'s: pulselessness, pallor, paresthesia, pain, paralysis, prostration) [6].

"Yellow flag" signs (Soft sign) (Fig. 10.2) are a history of arterial bleading at the scene or in transit, proximity of a penetrating wound or blunt injury to an artery, a small nonpulsatile hematoma over an artery or a neurologic deficit originating in a nerve adjacent to a named artery [6].

Every examination of the injured extremity should include the check of the peripherial pulses (A. radialis and A. ulnaris). The loss or diminishing of peripherial pulses is a serious sign for a malperfusion of the forearm. Even if there is a total disruption of the brachial artery a peripheral pulse might still be palpable [1]. A further symptom of a vascular injury could be a rapid progressive swelling of the elbow region as sign of a hematoma caused by a ruptured vessel. A cold and pale skin of the forearm or a delayed capillary refill can be a sign of the malperfusion of the upper limb.

If there is the smallest hint of a vascular injury a vascular specialist should be consulted. After the physical examination, a Doppler ultrasound is recommended. A monophasic or biphasic signal could be a sign for an insufficient perfusion and if available a duplex ultrasound should follow. One of the following examinations should be performed:

- Ankle or Brachial/Brachial Index (ABI or BBI = systolic blood pressure in extremity distal to the area of injury divided through thesystolic blood pressure in brachial artery of uninjured upper extremity.
- Arterial Pressure Index (API = Doppler arterial pressure distal to injury/divided through the Doppler arterial pressure from the uninvolved upper extremity [6, 7].

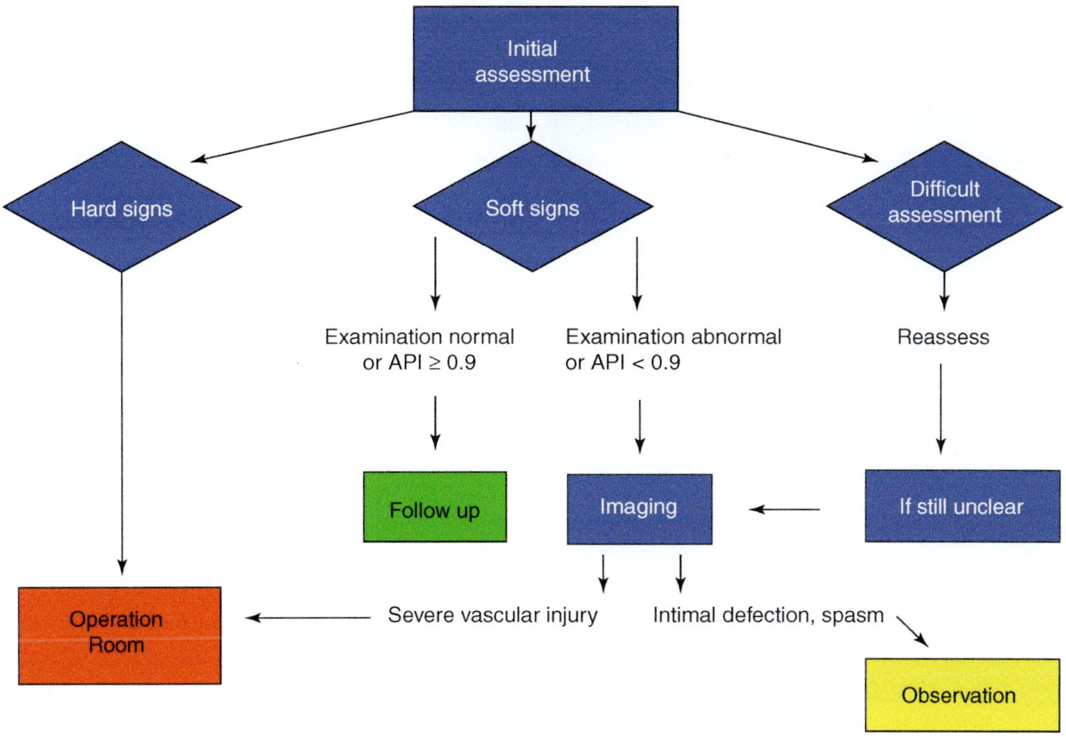

Fig. 10.2 Algorithm for evaluation of patient with suspected peripheral vascular injury. (Feliciano et al. 2011, modified by H. Wendorff 2017)

- If the ABI/API is below 0.9 a further diagnostic imaging is needed.

With the duplex/colour coded ultrasound examination, the continuity, injury or a disruption of the vessels can be approved. The duplex ultrasound has an excellent accuracy in assessing arterial injuries. The sensitivity is reported to reach 100% and the specifity exceeds 95% [8–12]. The quality and availability of the ultrasound depends on special trained technicians or vascular surgeons.

If no ultrasound is available or the situation remains unclear, a CT-Angiography (CTA) or a conventional angiography of the upper extremity is necessary [13]. Because these leads to a delay in treatment, this increases the complication rate by 1–4% (Fig. 10.3).

After the initial assessment of the vascular system, further controls are mandatory to check the status of the vascular perfusion and avoid to miss a forsening which might leds to severe damages due to hypoxia or structural changes [1].

Injury Pattern and Surgery Related Anatomy

The majority of elbow traumas are closed and the dislocation is posterior, but a small percentage are either anterior dislocations or open limb fractures [14]. Depending on the kind of trauma, a direct injury by bone fragments creates a penetrating vessel injury, were as on the otherside a stretching, overstreching or rupturing by the dislocated joint produces a blunt vessel injury.

Most commonly the transection is probably caused by a quick posterior movement of the unflexible bicipital aponeurosis, which is above the artery [15]. But as it is described, traumatic brachial artery rupture can already occur just by

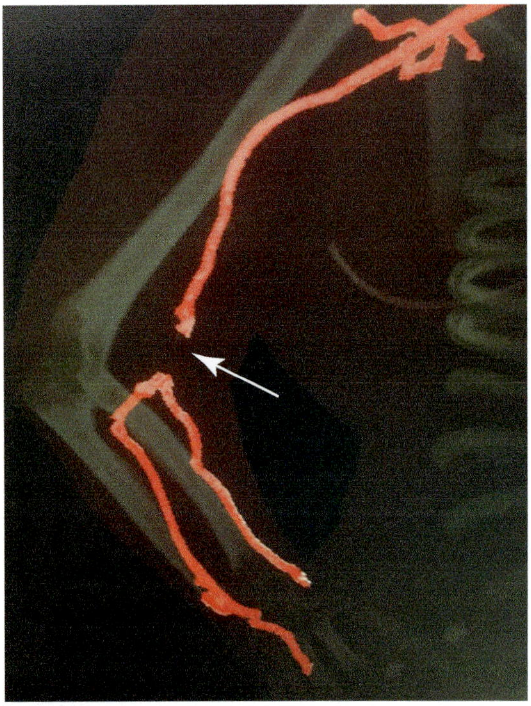

Fig. 10.3 CT-Angiography left upper extremity (discontinuated brachial artery (Arrow))

hyperextension of the elbow without accompanying luxation [16].

In the case of a posterior luxation, the brachial artery, which is located at the medial edge of the brachial biceps, dislocates together with the median nerve more ventrally and is then consecutively injured through the aponeurosis, which moves in the opposite direction, as it is still fixed to the bone [17].

A great number of collaterals (Fig. 10.4), so called radial recurrent artery, anterior and posterior ulnar recurrent artery, inferior and superior ulnar collateral artery, can compensate the disrupted brachial artery.

Therapeutic Options

Non-operative Treatment

Before the Korean War in the years 1950–1953 the accepted therapeutic management of major brachial artery injuries consistet out of ligation of the injured vessel, relying on the collateral circulation [18]. The problem was, that if the collateral circulation wasn't sufficient enough or was disrupted as well, the malperfusion of the forearm led to a gangrene or even an amputation [19].

Today each injury of the brachial artery should be examined by a vascular specialist and should then underwent open surgery if necessary. In isolated cases an endovascular approach is feasible but requires a safe passage of a guidewire through the injured vessel to restore distal perfusion [20]. The longterm patency of endovascular treatment in the brachial artery is unknown [21], in the literature only some case reports are reported [20, 22]. If an endovascular approach is favored, it should be done in a hybrid OR to be able to convert when necessary and treat associated injuries as well [20].

Exeptions are for example no “Redflag” sign [6] for a vessel injury, in combination with palpable peripheral pulses and good Doppler signals (triphasic) [14].

In the case of a decision for non-operative treatment it is recommended to reevaluate the perfusion in frequent intervals. A permanent pulse oximetry on the injured extremity can help to identify a late worsening of the perfusion state, which especially can occur in patients with grade 2 blunt vascular injury (according to the Vollmar classification), which is often missed on the initial physical examination.

Surgical Treatment

An absolute indication for open surgery, is the case of an open fracture in the elbow region. Hereby the vessels should be extensively examined. Also in case of an closed trauma with an suspected vascular injury an open surgery by a vascular surgeon is necessary. The surgeon should ideally wear a magnification loupe or should use the operating microscope. Beside the usual instruments special vascular instrument should be available (retractors, vascular scissors, vascular forceps, fine-tipped needle holders, vessel loops, Fogarty ballons with stopcocks,

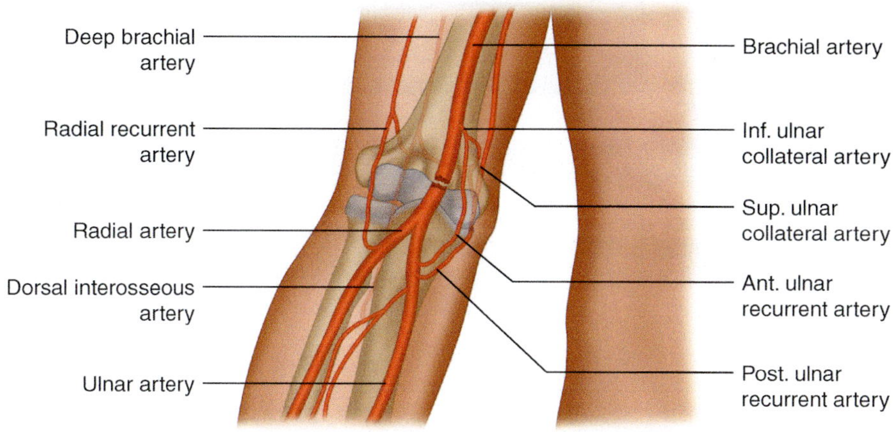

Fig. 10.4 Arterial collateral circulation around the elbow. (Marcheix et al. [15])

unfractionated heparin solution and contrast agent for the angiography) [23]. The skin disinfection of the injured upper extremity should include the whole arm because of the proximal and distal control of the potential injured brachial artery and to check the perfusion of the hand and the peripheral pulses during surgery [4, 24].

To expose the brachial artery proximal and distal to the elbow, a "lazy S" skin incision should be used [25]. It is important to dissect far enough proximal and distal to control the inflow, the backbleeding as well as bleeding out of collaterals when exploring the injured region [25, 26]. After exposing the vessels vascular occlusion should be done by applying special vascular clamps (DeBakey, Dardik, Bulldog, Yasargil), block catheters orelastic vessel loops. Then the further exploration should be done by removing the hematoma which helps to better identify the anatomic structures. This can be difficult depending of the degree of damage (Fig. 10.5).

For the management of the vessel repair Feliciano et al. created 2013 an algorithm (Fig. 10.6).

Small lacerations can be repaired by lateral angiorrhaphy with 5/0 or 6/0 polypropylene sutures (transversely) [24]. If it is foreseeable, that the suture generates a significant stenosis, primarily a vein patch should be done. If the artery is disrupted completely and the ends of the artery are not strongly destructed, a direct end-to-end anastomosis is possible. If this would leds to tension on the ends or in the case of segmental loss of the artery, an autogenous reversed vein graft interposition is necessary (Fig. 10.7). This could be harvested for example from the same arm (e.g. basilic or cephalic vein) or an uninjured leg (great or small saphenous vein).

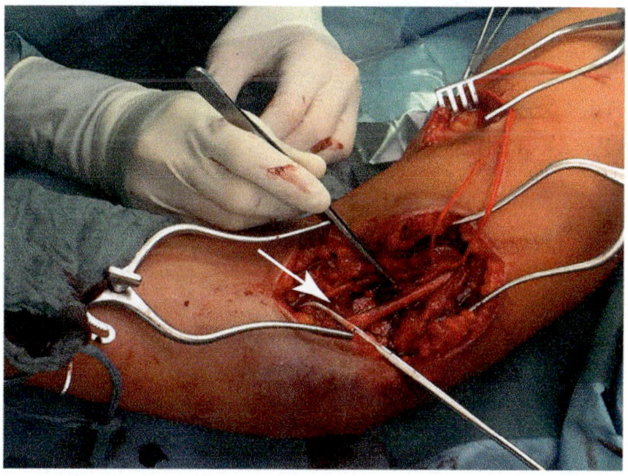

Fig. 10.5 Intraoperative exploration of the lacerated brachial artery; The proximal brachial artery is marked by a red vessel-loop, the distal end is tagged by an arrow and the median nerve is conserved

Alternatively if autologous veins are not available, a PTFE (polytetrafluorethylene) graft can be used. The long-term patency of PTFE grafts is significantly shorter compared to vein grafts [27].

If the soft tissue loss is to heavy, a muscle flap should be transposed to cover to neurovascular bundle. If this is not possible, an extraanatomic bypass should be considered early [28].

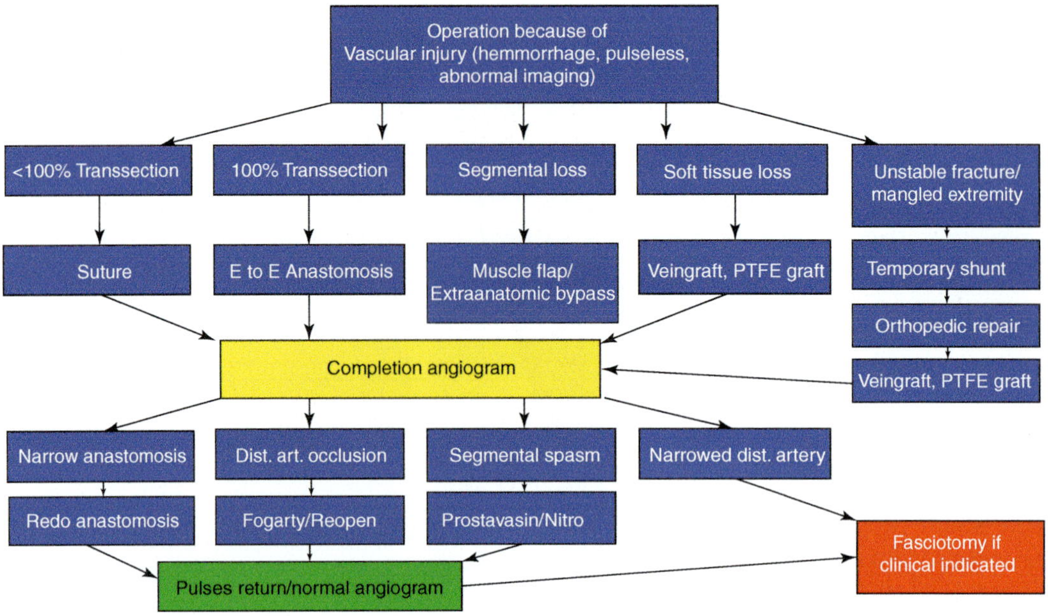

Fig. 10.6 Management algorithm for peripheral vascular injuries. (Feliciano et al. 2013, modified by H. Wendorff 2017)

A major complication after longer extremity ischemia and consecutive revascularization is a compartment syndrome. Therefor a prophylactic fasciotomia of the forearm might be necessary, depends on the swelling or on the severity of the ischemia.

At the end a completion angiography should be done to confirm a good result of the reconstruction and to identify early technical problems or rest thrombus in the arteries [23, 24, 29, 30] (Fig. 10.8).

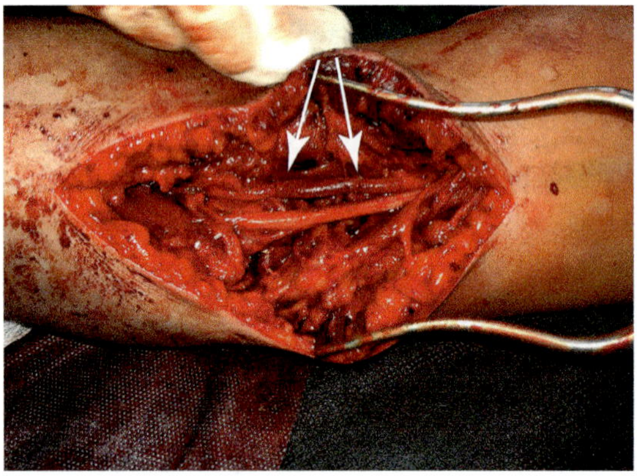

Fig. 10.7 Vein-Interposition with median cubital vein (prox. and distal anastomosis are tagged by an arrow)

Postoperative Care

Postoperative it is important to frequently examine the perfusion of the revascularized extremity to detect a further worsening of blood circulation at an early. The examination should include frequent test of the peripherial pulses as well as the sensibility of the forearm. If the patient requires intensive or intermediate care a pulse oximetry should be used to assess the extremity perfusion. An adequate infusion therapy is as important as the administration of an antiplatelet drug (ASS or Clopidogrel for a minimum of 3 month). Wound assessment should be done every day.

Four to six weeks after the revascularization an examination by a vascular surgeon including a duplex ultrasound should take place to evaluate the vascular reconstruction.

If there are any problems concerning the perfusion of the forearm a vascular specialist should immediately be consulted.

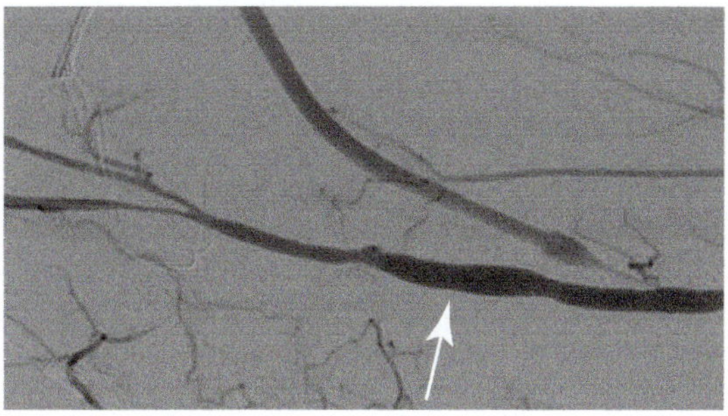

Fig. 10.8 Completion angiography after vein-interposition (Arrow)

Outcomes and Complications

Concerning, that only a small number of published cases exist, the overall outcome of patients receiving vascular repair after elbow trauma was satisfactory [3]. An analysis of nine cases done by Ayel et al. showed, that only one patient had a secondary thrombosis of the vascular graft, which required re-do surgery. All other patients (89%) had no complications related to the vascular reconstruction at a minimum of 2 years' follow up [17].

As already mentioned above, one of the most common complication beside the occlusion of the vascular graft is the development of a **compartment syndrome** [31–34]. The signs for the compartment syndrome are severe pain (particularly pressure pain, pain with passive stretch of the wrist and digits) [35, 36] and neurological deficiency (paresthesia) [37], they are frequently absent or masked in trauma patients because of refracting injuries and/or an altered mental status [24]. The key physical findings are disproportionate pain to the associated trauma and pain on passive movement of the muscles of the involved compartments. The real incidence of clinical relevant compartment syndrome after modern extremity vascular injury is unknown because of the common use of prophylactic fasciotomies [24, 25].

A prophylactic fasciotomy after arterial revascularization especially in combination with a dislocation or fracture can prevent a compartment syndrome and therefore its benefits clearly outweights the complications (wound healing, additional operative procedure) [38]. The fasciotomy of the forearm should particularly be performed in cases of late revascularization or complete or severe ischemia [17]. The skin incision should be done on the ventral side of the forearm in a straight line from the elbow region to the wrist joint [36]. The fasciotomy incisions should be executed to volar and dorsal faces of forearm [37] and should include the separation of the carpal tunnel to avoid compartment syndrome of the hand [36]. After the fasciotomy and the load removal of the muscle compartment, the wound should be covered with artificial skin (Epigard®, Orthomed Medizintechnik GmbH) and should be closed after a few days of detumescence [36].

References

1. Lutter C, Pfefferkorn R, Schoeffl V. Arterial damages in acute elbow dislocations: which diagnostic tests are required? BMJ Case Rep. 2016;2016:1–3.
2. Sparks SR, DeLaRosa J, Bergan JJ, Hoyt DB, Owens EL. Arterial injury in uncomplicated upper extremity dislocations. Ann Vasc Surg. 2000;14(2):110–3.
3. Endean ED, Veldenz HC, Schwarcz TH, Hyde GL. Recognition of arterial injury in elbow dislocation. J Vasc Surg. 1992;16(3):402–6.
4. Feliciano D. Evaluation and treatment of vascular injuries. In: Skeletal trauma basic science, management, and reconstruction. 4th ed. Philadelphia: Elsevier Saunders; 2009. p. 323–40.
5. Siebenlist S, Reeps C, Kraus T, Martetschlager F, Schmitt A, Stockle U, et al. Brachial artery transection caused by closed elbow dislocation in a mature in-line skater: a case report with review of the literature. Knee Surg Sports Traumatol Arthrosc Off J ESSKA. 2010;18(12):1667–70.
6. Feliciano DV, Moore FA, Moore EE, West MA, Davis JW, Cocanour CS, et al. Evaluation and management of peripheral vascular injury. Part 1. Western Trauma Association/critical decisions in trauma. J Trauma. 2011;70(6):1551–6.
7. Lynch K, Johansen K. Can Doppler pressure measurement replace "exclusion" arteriography in the diagnosis of occult extremity arterial trauma? Ann Surg. 1991;214(6):737–41.
8. Knudson MM, Lewis FR, Atkinson K, Neuhaus A. The role of duplex ultrasound arterial imaging in patients with penetrating extremity trauma. Arch Surg (Chicago, Ill: 1960). 1993;128(9):1033–7; discussion 1037–8.
9. Bynoe RP, Miles WS, Bell RM, Greenwold DR, Sessions G, Haynes JL, et al. Noninvasive diagnosis of vascular trauma by duplex ultrasonography. J Vasc Surg. 1991;14(3):346–52.
10. Fry WR, Smith RS, Sayers DV, Henderson VJ, Morabito DJ, Tsoi EK, et al. The success of duplex

ultrasonographic scanning in diagnosis of extremity vascular proximity trauma. Arch Surg (Chicago, Ill: 1960). 1993;128(12):1368–72.
11. Gagne PJ, Cone JB, McFarland D, Troillett R, Bitzer LG, Vitti MJ, et al. Proximity penetrating extremity trauma: the role of duplex ultrasound in the detection of occult venous injuries. J Trauma. 1995;39(6):1157–63.
12. Valentini MB, Farsetti P, Martinelli O, Laurito A, Ippolito E. The value of ultrasonic diagnosis in the management of vascular complications of supracondylar fractures of the humerus in children. Bone Joint J. 2013;95(5):694–8.
13. Halvorson JJ, Anz A, Langfitt M, Deonanan JK, Scott A, Teasdall RD, et al. Vascular injury associated with extremity trauma: initial diagnosis and management. J Am Acad Orthop Surg. 2011;19(8):495–504.
14. Grimer RJ, Brooks S. Brachial artery damage accompanying closed posterior dislocation of the elbow. J Bone Joint Surg. 1985;67(3):378–81.
15. Marcheix B, Chaufour X, Ayel J, Hollington L, Mansat P, Barret A, et al. Transection of the brachial artery after closed posterior elbow dislocation. J Vasc Surg. 2005;42(6):1230–2.
16. Jeyaretna DS, Butler M, David HG, Walker AJ. A case of elbow hyperextension leading to complete brachial artery rupture. World J Emerg Surg. 2007;2:6.
17. Ayel JE, Bonnevialle N, Lafosse JM, Pidhorz L, Al Homsy M, Mansat P, et al. Acute elbow dislocation with arterial rupture. Analysis of nine cases. Orthop Traumatol Surg Res. 2009;95(5):343–51.
18. Debakey ME, Simeone FA. Battle injuries of the arteries in world war II : an analysis of 2,471 cases. Ann Surg. 1946;123(4):534–79.
19. Ebong W. Gangrene complicating closed posterior dislocation of the elbow. Int Surg. 1978;63(1):44–5.
20. Smeets R, Ryckx A, Krasznai A, Sikkink C, Bouwman L. Endovascular treatment of blunt traumatic injury to the brachial Arterv: case report and review of the literature. Clin Med Rev Case Rep. 2017;4(8):179.
21. Johnson CA. Endovascular management of peripheral vascular trauma. Semin Interv Radiol. 2010;27(1):38–43.
22. Pin R. Endovascular repair of a transected proximal brachial artery. Endovasc Today. 2012;11(4):34–7.
23. Feliciano DV, Moore EE, West MA, Moore FA, Davis JW, Cocanour CS, et al. Western trauma association critical decisions in trauma: evaluation and management of peripheral vascular injury, part II. J Trauma Acute Care Surg. 2013;75(3):391–7.
24. Mavrogenis AF, Panagopoulos GN, Kokkalis ZT, Koulouvaris P, Megaloikonomos PD, Igoumenou V, et al. Vascular injury in orthopedic trauma. Orthopedics. 2016;39(4):249–59.
25. Kauvar DSK, Kraiss LW. Vascular trauma: extremity. In: Rutherford's vascular surgery. Philadelphia: Elsevier; 2014. p. 2485–500.
26. Feliciano DV. Management of peripheral arterial injury. Curr Opin Crit Care. 2010;16(6):602–8.
27. Feliciano DV, Mattox KL, Graham JM, Bitondo CG. Five-year experience with PTFE grafts in vascular wounds. J Trauma Acute Care Surg. 1985;25(1):71.
28. Feliciano DV. Heroic procedures in vascular injury management: the role of extra-anatomic bypasses. Surg Clin. 2002;82(1):115–24.
29. Kurtoglu M, Yanar H, Taviloglu K, Sivrikoz E, Plevin R, Aksoy M. Serious lower extremity venous injury management with ligation: prospective overview of 63 patients. Am Surg. 2007;73(10):1039–43.
30. Parry NG, Feliciano DV, Burke RM, Cava RA, Nicholas JM, Dente CJ, et al. Management and short-term patency of lower extremity venous injuries with various repairs. Am J Surg. 2003;186(6):631–5.
31. Branco BC, Inaba K, Barmparas G, Schnüriger B, Lustenberger T, Talving P, et al. Incidence and predictors for the need for fasciotomy after extremity trauma: a 10-year review in a mature level I trauma Centre. Injury. 2011;42(10):1157–63.
32. Sheridan GW, Matsen FA 3rd. Fasciotomy in the treatment of the acute compartment syndrome. J Bone Joint Surg Am. 1976;58(1):112–5.
33. Ellis H. Disabilities after tibial shaft fractures; with special reference to Volkmann's ischaemic contracture. J Bone Joint Surg Br. 1958;40-b(2):190–7.
34. Muehlbacher J, Klinger M. Das Kompartmentsyndrom des Unterschenkels - Diagnostik und Therapie. Zeitschrift fuer Gefaessmedizin. 2013;10(2):7–14.
35. Kistler JM, Ilyas AM, Thoder JJ. Forearm compartment syndrome: evaluation and management. Hand Clin. 2018;34(1):53–60.
36. Berdel P, Gravius S, Goldmann G, Pennekamp P, Oldenburg J, Seuser A, et al. Das muskuläre Kompartmentsyndrom am Unterarm bei Hemmkörperhämophilie. Hamostaseologie. 2008;28(4):45–9.
37. Sayar U, Özer T, Mataracı İ. Forearm compartment syndrome caused by reperfusion injury. Case Rep Vasc Med. 2014;2014:931410.
38. Farber A, Tan T-W, Hamburg NM, Kalish JA, Joglar F, Onigman T, et al. Early fasciotomy in patients with extremity vascular injury is associated with decreased risk of adverse limb outcomes: a review of the National Trauma Data Bank. Injury. 2012;43(9):1486–91.

Nerve Injury in Adults

11

Stephan Deiler and Helen Vester

Epidemiology of Nerve Injuries

Nerve injury is an uncommon complication of fractures and dislocations of the elbow. The assessment and treatment of nerve dysfunction after trauma around the elbow remains a challenging and controversial topic. The anatomic positions of the radial, median, and ulnar nerves and their major branches make them vulnerable at several sites (see Fig. 11.1a, b). This is the reason for the relationship between particular nerve injuries and fracture patterns, such as radial nerve paralysis and humerus shaft fracture. Posterior interosseus nerve injury with Monteggia fracture dislocation [1] and/or anterior interosseus nerve injuries with elbow dislocation [1].

When recognized as a paralysis after elbow trauma, it is not always clear how severe the nerve injury may be, although most lower energy injuries are fully recoverable. Although the time frame to intervention remains controversial for specific injuries, longstanding dysfunction necessitates surgical exploration and either neurolysis, transposition, repair, and/or reconstruction with tendon transfers. Considerable controversy remains regarding the need for early exploration in closed humeral shaft or supracondylar fractures and the role of ulnar nerve transposition after elbow trauma.

Ulnar neuropathy is associated with fractures of the distal humerus in up to 50% of patients [2–4]. This prevalence of injury is multifactorial and the result of the proximity of the nerve to the injury zone, handling of the nerve during surgical intervention, or postoperative scarring around the implants and the surgical site [5].

Classification of Nerve Injuries

Nerve injuries are commonly classified according to the Sunderland classification. The mildest injuries are *neurapraxias* (Sunderland grade 1), which involve dysfunction without nerve sheath disruption [6–8]. The nerve velocities in this type of injury may be normal or may slow 1–3 weeks after injury. Subsequent electromyography (EMG) studies may show recruitment of muscles units and fibres [7].

Sunderland grade 2, also called *axonotmesis* is the result of internal nerve fibre damage, which results in complete Wallerian degeneration [7, 8]. These may be secondary to stretch injury [9]. However, the endoneurium remains intact, which

S. Deiler (✉) · H. Vester
Interdicsiplinary Center of Hands (IHZ), Clinic and Polyclinic for Trauma Surgery and Orthopedics, Munich, Germany
e-mail: Stephan.Deiler@mri.tum.de

P. Biberthaler et al. (eds.), *Acute Elbow Trauma*, Strategies in Fracture Treatments,
https://doi.org/10.1007/978-3-319-97850-5_11

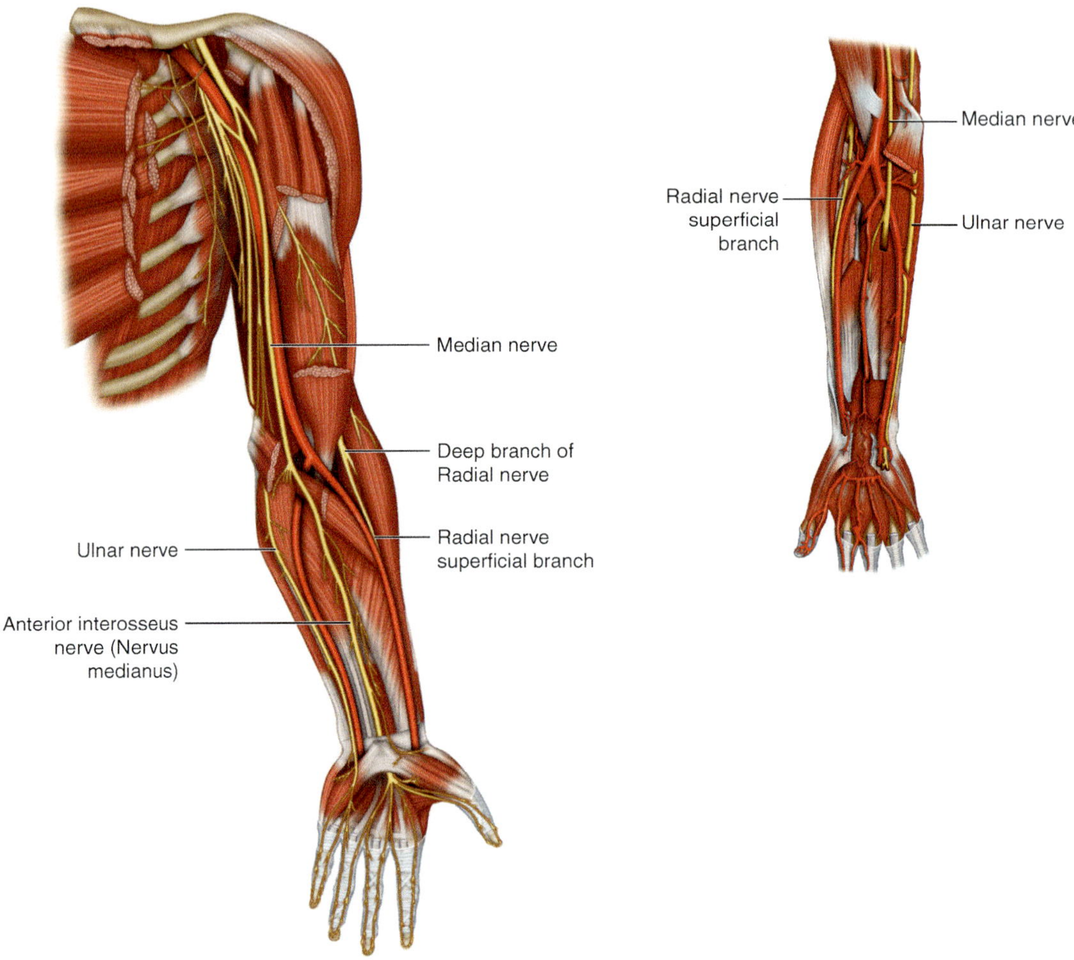

Fig. 11.1 Anatomy of the peripheral nerves. (**a**, **b**) Depict the nerves of the upper limb. Exact anatomic knowledge is mandatory for a surgical approach and understanding of certain patterns of injury or nerve deficiency

helps guiding the regenerating fibres to the distal end fibres [8]. Up to 7 days after trauma, the distal nerve conduction velocities may be normal with denervation occurring at 2–5 weeks and re-innervation at 6–8 weeks after injury [8, 7]. These two categories however have a good to excellent prognosis for spontaneous resolution [6, 8, 10]. Injuries according to Sunderland grade 3–5 are classifies as *neurotmesis.* They involve a complete division of the nerve and do require surgical intervention for recovery of function [8, 10]. In the majority of cases, injuries of nerves about the elbow are grade 1 or 2 after Sunderland and occur mostly after transient stretching or compression from fracture fragments, tissue oedema or haematoma [8, 10].

Fractures can typically lead to *neurapraxia,* while *axonotmesis* or *neurotmesis* are more likely a consequence of fracture fragment dislocation [7]. Blunt trauma typically results in *axonotmesis* or *neurapraxia* [11] (see Table 11.1 [12, 13]).

Table 11.1 Sunderland and Seddon classification [12, 13]

Type 1	Conduction block (neurapraxia)
Type 2	Axonal injury (axonotmesis)
Type 3	Type 2 + Endoneurium injury
Type 4	Type 3 + Perineurium injury
Type 5	Type 4 + Epineurium injury (neurotmesis)

This table depicts the classification of nerve injuries according to the Sunderland and Seddon classifications. Both classifications overlap. While Seddon classified nerve injuries into three different categories: neurapraxia, axonotmesis, and neurotmesis; Sunderland expanded Seddon's axonotmetic category, for a total of five degrees of nerve injury. Basic knowledge of the different degrees of nerve injury is mandatory to understand the need for observation in some patients and for surgical intervention in others

Diagnosis, Evaluation and Therapy of Nerve Injuries

A complete and careful physical examination and clinical history are eminent for correct diagnosis and accurate assessment of nerve injury, which is essential for initiation of the correct therapy [6, 8, 14]. Radiographic, nerve conduction and EMG studies may be helpful but most authors recommend waiting to obtain EMG studies for at least 3–4 weeks after injury [14]. Earlier EMG studies typically only show a conduction block at the injury segment but may fail to differentiate between neurapraxia and axonal loss. Therefore, waiting a minimum of 3–4 weeks after injury to obtain EMG studies maximises diagnostic accuracy in terms of localization and degree of injury [8, 11].

However, some authors also advocate using EMG early on to differentiate neurapraxic injuries from more severe lesions as sometimes fibrillation potentials (suggesting a Wallerian degeneration, which means an axonal loss) may be seen as early as 10 days after injury [6]. Regarding nerve injury treatment there are several possibilities ranging from observation, exploration and neurolysis, or excision of the injured segment with nerve grafting, nerve transfers, or tendon transfers [6, 14, 15 16] (Fig. 11.2). No matter which definite treatment for the nerve injury is chosen, it is eminent to take supportive care of the patient in the meantime. Fracture management, optimizing conditions for soft tissue healing, prevention of infections and maintaining joint mobility are crucial steps at every stage of nerve injury management [11]. Moreover, it is eminent to protect insensate skin from further injury [15].

In case of a traumatic peripheral nerve laceration, an immediate end- to-end repair of the nerve is indicated [6]. Sometimes, nerve ends are badly contused or otherwise damaged, so that a delay of 2–3 weeks can be discussed to allow tissue demarcation to occur with subsequent primary or nerve graft repair [6, 17]. In general, a primary end-to-end suture repair under minimal tension is clearly preferred, however, if a large structural gap is present then a nerve graft may be required [6]. For this nerve graft, the sural nerve or the lateral antebrachial or medial antebrachial cutaneous nerve can be used [6].

In case of proximal nerve injuries with a great distance to the corresponding muscle, unreconstructable segmental nerve tissue loss or brachial plexus avulsion injuries, a nerve transfer may be indicated [16]. A nerve transfer includes complex rerouting of active nerves to the denervated end organ, including transfer of proximal trunks from normal nerves to the distal stumps of the injured nerve. Afterwards, for cortical remapping, a complex and complicated rehabilitation course is required [15].

It is known that the motor end plates become refractory to re-innervation between 15 and 18 months in adults [16]. As the nerve regeneration after repair proceeds generally at a rate of about 1 mm per day [15], the time frame in which the denervated muscle can be successfully re-innervated after nerve repair can be calculated. Irreversible muscle atrophy occurs probably after 18 months, therefore this is the time frame in which the regenerated nerve must reach the target muscle. Thus, for successful nerve reconstruction, the sum of the duration from denervation to repair in months plus the distance from the site of injury to the target muscle should be less than 18 [16].

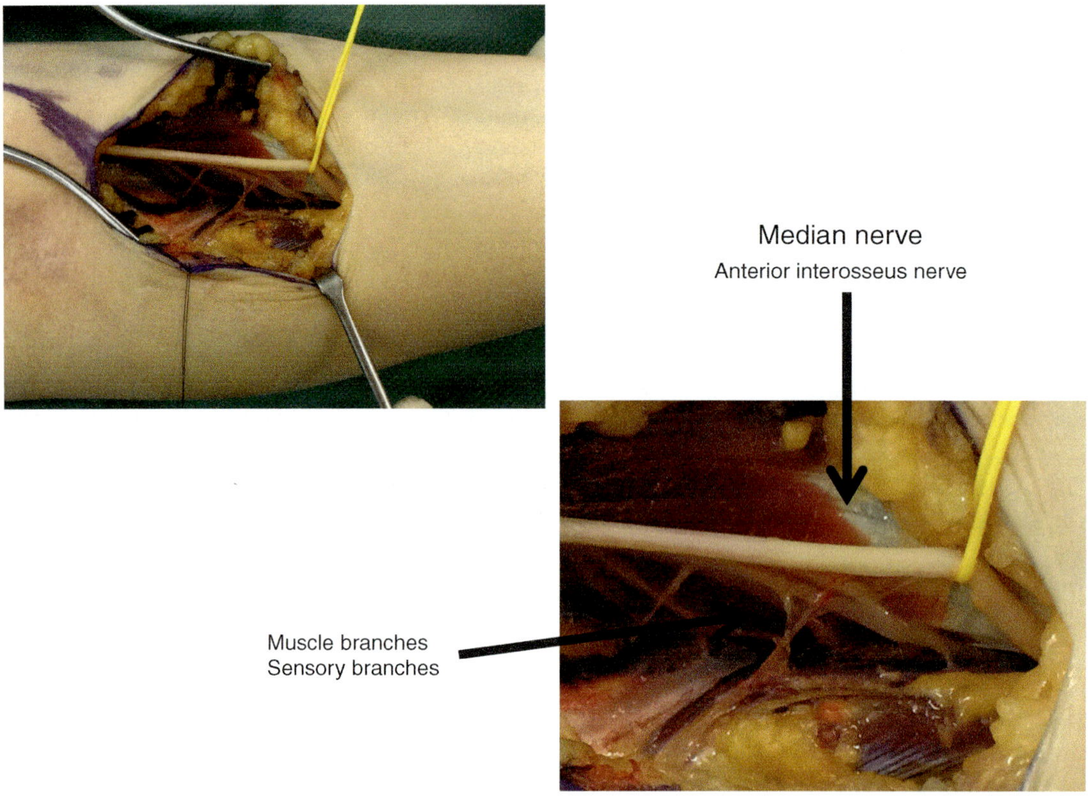

Fig. 11.2 Clinical aspect of the median nerve during surgical exploration at the elbow. This patient has been suffering from an AIN nerve palsy for several months without signs of recovery. Therefore a surgical exploration was indicated. During surgery no signs of nerve injury could be found, therefore we diagnosed a neurapraxia and proceeded with conservative treatment and observation

For evaluation of the nerve function return several signs may be helpful on clinical evaluation [18]. The examination of motor function and strength [19] is of course obligatory. Sweating may be seen without sensory return but return of sensation is rarely seen without preceding or accompanying return of sweating. Other useful signs are the monitoring of the vibratory sensation and the two point discrimination [18].

Nerve Injuries After Fractures

Up to 80–90% of the upper limb nerve injuries are caused by fractures [7]. However, nearly all of these nerve injuries (86–100%) in every age group are neurapraxias which means that no surgical intervention is necessary as they recover spontaneously within 2–6 months [6–8]. Thus, observation for 6 months, followed by electrodiagnostic studies to facilitate a decision about surgery is the recommended treatment [8]. However, some particular nerve palsies have been found to be more common with certain elbow injuries [7, 8].

Radial Nerve Injury/Palsy with Fractures of the Humerus Shaft

Radial nerve palsy after fractures of the humerus is the most common nerve lesion in long bone fracture, the most common cause being diaphyseal humerus shaft fractures [20–22] which accounts for approximately 3% of all orthopaedic injuries [23–26]. Its relationship to the radial nerve injury is due to the anatomic position of the nerve in the transition from the middle to the distal third of the humerus [24, 27, 28].

The incidence of radial nerve injury associated with diaphyseal humerus fracture is cited in the literature between 11% and 18%, indicating car accidents as the leading cause, mainly young men and older women represent the affected population [23, 26].

The classic clinical symptoms of the radial nerve palsy are the inability to extend the wrist, loss of extension of the fingers in the metacarpophalangeal joints and inability to extend and abduct the thumb. This leads to the typical known wrist-drop deformity which represents a significant functional damage to the hand, since the inability to extend and stabilize the wrist prevents proper use of extrinsic flexors for hand closing, thus, weakening and lowering the grip and diminishing coordination.

In spite of permanent improvement of therapeutic strategies for a better patient outcome, there is still a controversy regarding the best treatment and time point of radial nerve palsy. Noncontroversial indications for early exploration include: fractures with unacceptable alignment or secondary dislocation after closed treatment, open fractures, fractures with associated vascular injuries and multiple limb involvement in patients with polytrauma. So far, the literature remains indecisive about closed fractures that can be treated conservatively.

However, early exploration of the radial nerve seems to be advantageous in some points. It is technically easier and safer than the delayed procedure. Direct examination of the nerve clarifies the diagnosis and the extent of the lesion. By early stabilization of the fracture the risk of the nerve being trapped by scar tissue and callus can be reduced. Reduction of the open fracture helps to minimize the risk of further damage to the nerve from mobile bone ends [29–32].

The opponents of early exploration claim high rates of spontaneous recovery and have advised a policy of expectancy [10, 33, 34], for prevention of unnecessary complications attendant on exploration. They argument that the real extent of the neurilemmal sheath damage cannot be stated immediately but it needs some time until the extent of nerve damage can be defined, which makes repair easier. Moreover, it is more comfortable to treat the nerve when the fracture is healed. However, these studies are uncontrolled retrospective case series, mostly with only small number of patients [31]. Noaman et al. recommend early radial nerve exploration (within the first 2 weeks) in patients with open fractures of humerus with radial nerve injury, fractures of distal third of humerus either transverse or oblique and in postreduction radial nerve injury [35]. On exploration often nerve compression at the intermuscular septum, an entrapment in the fracture site or even loss of its continuity can be found. Some authors have also described a negative exploration [31].

Regarding the injury or irritation of the nerve, different treatment options are given. If the nerve is entrapped in the muscle or by the fracture, a neurolysis is indicated, if the nerve is cut in two or partially injured, epineurorrhaphy needs to be performed. If epineural radial nerve repair cannot be performed primarily or secondarily due to a defect in the nerve, a nerve graft is needed. In the severe and rare case of a total avulsion of the radial nerve from the posterior cord, a first-intention tendon transfer can be performed.

Monteggia Lesion and Nerve Injury

Monteggia fractures are classified according the Bado classification [36]. It is a fracture of the proximal third of the ulna with a concomitant anterior dislocation of the radial head. The radial nerve can be involved in a Monteggia lesion by the fracture dislocation. After having given off the ramus superficialis with motor and cutaneous sensory fibres, the nerve continues in ramus profundus, giving off motor branches to the extensor carpi radialis brevis and supinator muscles. The ramus profundus enters the supinator proximal the neck of the radius. After emerging from the supinator it gives off branches to the extensor muscles and the abductor pollicis longus and the extensor pollicis longus and brevis. In 30% a fibrous arch can be found at the muscle insertion, which helds the nerve tight to the bone. Compressions of the nerve often occur at this point [37].

There has been great variation in the reported incidence of nerve injury and the degree of spontaneous recovery after Monteggia fractures of the elbow. Most large series mix pediatric and adult patients and various types of Monteggia fractures and their equivalents.

Several mechanisms of traumatic neuropathies of the radial and ulnar nerves that are associated with Monteggia lesions have been documented and discussed. Some described the nerve lesion following Monteggia fracture as the result of a direct trauma or a compression of the nerve [38], an entrapment between the radius and ulna, a stretching of the nerve due to the dislocation of the radial head, a delayed palsy as the result of an old unreduced radial head and displacement of the nerve around the radial neck during attempted closed reduction [39]. Patients with a neuropathy of the anterior interosseus nerve present with partial or total paralysis of the flexor pollicis longus, the flexor digitorum to the index finger, and the pronator quadratus, with no loss of sensation [40]. There are also a few cases reported with higher ulnar nerve lesions and posterior interosseous nerve palsy [41]. In two cases, the nerve was explored at the elbow and a soft pseudoneuroma proximal to the site of constriction between the two heads of the flexor carpi ulnaris could be detected. In general, the neurologic lesions after Monteggia resolve spontaneously and Givon and other authors suggested that the nerves should be explored only in cases of irreducible dislocation [41, 42]. Some authors recommend exploration at 12 weeks if no sign of spontaneous recovery is present [41]. Moreover, an open reduction and exploration of the posterior interosseus nerve may be necessary in case of chronic dislocation or subluxation of the radial head [8].

Dislocation of the Elbow and Nerve Injury

Although nerve injury after elbow dislocation is well described, the true incidence can only be estimated about 14%. The true incidence remains elusive as the literature is full of case reports and series but they combine children with adults and simple dislocation with fracture and/or dislocation [43–45]. The most common injury seems to be an ulnar nerve neurapraxia that spontaneously resolves after closed reduction [7, 8]. Usually, the median nerve, radial nerve, or posterior interosseus nerve are affected only in rare cases [8, 16, 44]. However, in general, these nerve lesions recover spontaneously. There are a few cases reported in the literature with unfavourable outcomes after closed elbow dislocation and ulnar nerve lesions like persistent dysesthesia and two patients out of 1546 needed a nerve transposition [42, 44].

Summary

Nerve injury is an uncommon complication of fractures and dislocations of the elbow. However, the anatomic positions of the radial, median, and ulnar nerves and their major branches make them vulnerable at several sites. This is the reason for the relationship between particular nerve injuries and fracture patterns, such as radial nerve paralysis and humerus shaft fracture. Posterior interosseus nerve injury with Monteggia fracture dislocation and/or anterior interosseus nerve injuries with elbow dislocation. Nerve lesions are classified according to the Sunderland classification. Generally, nerve lesions after elbow trauma or closed elbow dislocations are neurapraxia or axonetmesis (Sunderland grade 1 or 2), with a good to excellent prognosis for spontaneous resolution. Therefore, in most cases injury represents contusion of the nerve and is managed adequately by observation and supportive measures alone. Noncontroversial indications for early exploration include: fractures with unacceptable alignment or secondary dislocation after closed treatment, open fractures, fractures with associated vascular injuries and multiple limb involvement in patients with polytrauma. Nevertheless, caution should be exercised when performing procedures in this region and a thorough knowledge and appreciation of the relevant neuroanatomy of this region is crucial.

In case of persisting nerve palsy after elbow trauma and conservative treatment for 3 months a surgical exploration is indicated. No matter which final treatment for the nerve palsy is indicated, these patients need close monitoring, physiotherapy and adequate support as nerve repair takes its time.

References

1. Adams JE, Steinmann SP. Nerve injuries about the elbow. The Journal of hand surgery. 2006;31(2):303–13.
2. McKee MD, Jupiter JB, Bosse G, Goodman L. Outcome of ulnar neurolysis during post-traumatic reconstruction of the elbow. J Bone Joint Surg. 1998;80(1):100–5.
3. Kundel K, Braun W, Wieberneit J, Ruter A. Intraarticular distal humerus fractures. Factors affecting functional outcome Clinical orthopaedics and related research. 1996;332:200–8.
4. Holdsworth BJ, Mossad MM. Fractures of the adult distal humerus. Elbow function after internal fixation. J Bone Joint Surg. 1990;72(3):362–5.
5. Wang KC, Shih HN, Hsu KY, Shih CH. Intercondylar fractures of the distal humerus: routine anterior subcutaneous transposition of the ulnar nerve in a posterior operative approach. J Trauma. 1994;36(6):770–3.
6. Grant GA, Goodkin R, Kliot M. Evaluation and surgical management of peripheral nerve problems. Neurosurgery. 1999;44(4):825–39; discussion 839–40.
7. Nelson AJ, Izzi JA, Green A, Weiss AP, Akelman E. Traumatic nerve injuries about the elbow. Orthop Clin North Am. 1999;30(1):91–4.
8. Ristic S, Strauch RJ, Rosenwasser MP. The assessment and treatment of nerve dysfunction after trauma around the elbow. Clin Orthop Relat Res. 2000;370:138–53.
9. Belin BM, Ball DJ, Langer JC, Bridge PM, Hagberg PK, Mackinnon SE. The effect of age on peripheral motor nerve function after crush injury in the rat. J Trauma. 1996;40(5):775–7.
10. Samardzic M, Grujicic D, Milinkovic ZB. Radial nerve lesions associated with fractures of the humeral shaft. Injury. 1990;21(4):220–2.
11. Thoder JJ, Kozin SH. Management principles to treat nerve loss after violent trauma to the upper extremity. Hand Clin. 1999;15(2):289–98, ix.
12. Sunderland S. A classification of peripheral nerve injuries producing loss of function. Brain. 1951;74(4):491–516.
13. Seddon H. Surgical disorders of the peripheral nerves. 2nd ed. New York: Churchill Livingstone; 1975.
14. Hirachi K, Kato H, Minami A, Kasashima T, Kaneda K. Clinical features and management of traumatic posterior interosseous nerve palsy. J Hand Surg Br. 1998;23(3):413–7.
15. Chiu DT, Ishii C. Management of peripheral nerve injuries. Orthop Clin North Am. 1986;17(3):365–73.
16. Nath RK, Mackinnon SE. Nerve transfers in the upper extremity. Hand Clin. 2000;16(1):131–9, ix.
17. Ring D, Chin K, Jupiter JB. Radial nerve palsy associated with high-energy humeral shaft fractures. The Journal of hand surgery. 2004;29(1):144–7.
18. Lovett WL, McCalla MA. Nerve injuries: management and rehabilitation. Orthop Clin North Am. 1983;14(4):767–78.
19. Vanderhooft E. Functional outcomes of nerve grafts for the upper and lower extremities. Hand Clin. 2000;16(1):93–104, ix.
20. Thomsen NO, Dahlin LB. Injury to the radial nerve caused by fracture of the humeral shaft: timing and neurobiological aspects related to treatment and diagnosis. Scand J Plast Reconstr Surg Hand Surg. 2007;41(4):153–7.
21. Lowe JB 3rd, Sen SK, Mackinnon SE. Current approach to radial nerve paralysis. Plast Reconstr Surg. 2002;110(4):1099–113.
22. Ciaramitaro P, Mondelli M, Logullo F, Grimaldi S, Battiston B, Sard A, et al. Traumatic peripheral nerve injuries: epidemiological findings, neuropathic pain and quality of life in 158 patients. J Peripher Nerv Syst. 2010;15(2):120–7.
23. Steffner RJ, Lee MA. Emerging concepts in upper extremity trauma: humeral shaft fractures. Orthop Clin North Am. 2013;44(1):21–33.
24. Spiguel AR, Steffner RJ. Humeral shaft fractures. Curr Rev Musculoskelet Med. 2012;5(3):177–83.
25. Mahabier KC, Vogels LM, Punt BJ, Roukema GR, Patka P, Van Lieshout EM. Humeral shaft fractures: retrospective results of non-operative and operative treatment of 186 patients. Injury. 2013;44(4):427–30.
26. Walker M, Palumbo B, Badman B, Brooks J, Van Gelderen J, Mighell M. Humeral shaft fractures: a review. J Shoulder Elbow Surg. 2011;20(5):833–44.
27. Chaudhry T, Noor S, Maher B, Bridger J. The surgical anatomy of the radial nerve and the triceps aponeurosis. Clin Anat. 2010;23(2):222–6.
28. Carlan D, Pratt J, Patterson JM, Weiland AJ, Boyer MI, Gelberman RH. The radial nerve in the brachium: an anatomic study in human cadavers. J Hand Surg. 2007;32(8):1177–82.
29. Packer JW, Foster RR, Garcia A, Grantham SA. The humeral fracture with radial nerve palsy: is exploration warranted? Clin Orthop Relat Res. 1972;88:34–8.
30. Holstein A, Lewis GM. Fractures of the Humerus with Radial-Nerve Paralysis. J Bone Joint Surg Am. 1963;45:1382–8.
31. Foster RJ, Swiontkowski MF, Bach AW, Sack JT. Radial nerve palsy caused by open humeral shaft fractures. The Journal of hand surgery. 1993;18(1):121–4.
32. Dabezies EJ, Banta CJ 2nd, Murphy CP, D'Ambrosia RD. Plate fixation of the humeral shaft for acute fractures, with and without radial nerve injuries. J Orthop Trauma. 1992;6(1):10–3.

33. Larsen LB, Barfred T. Radial nerve palsy after simple fracture of the humerus. Scand J Plast Reconstr Surg Hand Surg. 2000;34(4):363–6.
34. Amillo S, Barrios RH, Martinez-Peric R, Losada JI. Surgical treatment of the radial nerve lesions associated with fractures of the humerus. J Orthop Trauma. 1993;7(3):211–5.
35. Noaman H, Khalifa AR, El-Deen MA, Shiha A. Early surgical exploration of radial nerve injury associated with fracture shaft humerus. Microsurgery. 2008;28(8):635–42.
36. Bado JL. The Monteggia lesion. Clin Orthop Relat Res. 1967;50:71–86.
37. Jessing P. Monteggia lesions and their complicating nerve damage. Acta Orthop Scand. 1975;46(4):601–9.
38. Spar I. A neurologic complication following Monteggia fracture. Clin Orthop Relat Res. 1977;122:207–9.
39. Lichter RL, Jacobsen T. Tardy palsy of the posterior interosseous nerve with a Monteggia fracture. J Bone Joint Surg Am. 1975;57(1):124–5.
40. Engber WD, Keene JS. Anterior interosseous nerve palsy associated with a Monteggia fracture. A case report Clinical orthopaedics and related research. 1983;174:133–7.
41. Stein F, Grabias SL, Deffer PA. Nerve injuries complicating Monteggia lesions. J Bone Joint Surg Am. 1971;53(7):1432–6.
42. Galbraith KA, McCullough CJ. Acute nerve injury as a complication of closed fractures or dislocations of the elbow. Injury. 1979;11(2):159–64.
43. Cohen MS, Hastings H 2nd. Acute elbow dislocation: evaluation and management. J Am Acad Orthop Surg. 1998;6(1):15–23.
44. Mehlhoff TL, Noble PC, Bennett JB, Tullos HS. Simple dislocation of the elbow in the adult. Results after closed treatment. J Bone Joint Surg Am. 1988;70(2):244–9.
45. Webb S, Lourie J. Median nerve entrapment in an unreduced fracture-dislocation of the elbow: case report. P N G Med J. 1986;29(2):185–7.

Printed by Printforce, the Netherlands